東洋医学の英語を学ぶ
Medical English for Oriental Medicine

高木 久代　Hisayo Takagi
木村 研一　Kenichi Kimura
西村 甲　Ko Nishimura
高木 健　Ken Takagi

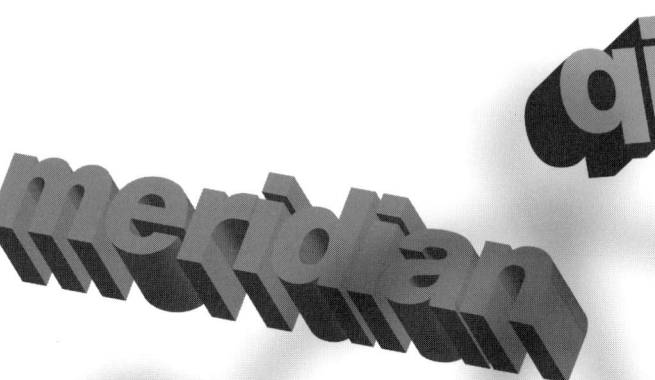

医歯薬出版株式会社

執筆一覧

執筆順

高木久代（鈴鹿医療科学大学・教授）
木村研一（関西医療大学・准教授）
西村　甲（伊勢慶友病院・小児科部長）
高木　健（鈴鹿医療科学大学・助教）

This book was originally published in Japanese under the title of：

TOUYOUIGAKU DE EIGO WO MANABU
(Medical English for Oriental Medicine)

TAKAGI, Hisayo et al.
　Professor,
　Suzuka University of Medical Science

© 2013 1st ed.

ISHIYAKU PUBLISHERS, INC.
　7-10, Honkomagome 1 chome, Bunkyo-ku,
　Tokyo 113-8612, Japan

はじめに
preface

　医療は変わりつつあります。医療の高度化と専門分化が進んだ結果、医療の主役は「チーム医療」へと変わりました。また、これからは「統合医療の時代」と言われるように、西洋医学に東洋医学など代替医療を合わせて治療にあたる新たな医療の試みが始まっています。特に慢性疾患治療に関しては、鍼灸師がチーム医療の一員として医療に関わることが期待されています。この代替医療や統合医療の流れは、日本ばかりではなく、アメリカ、カナダ、ドイツなど世界的に広がりつつあります。

　チーム医療に関わる人たちは、医療の高度化に対応していくため、最新の医療知識や技術が必要となりますが、医学や医療に関わる研究、論文、文献のほとんどは英語で書かれているため、英語能力は必要不可欠なものとなっています。

　本書は鍼灸を専門とする学生が、東洋医学と英語を同時に学習することを目指していますが、東洋医学を専門としない学生や社会人の方にも、本書を通して鍼灸、漢方、薬膳などの基礎を理解しながら英語を学んで頂けると思います。

【内容とその特徴】

　本書は「東洋医学の歴史」から始まり、鍼灸、ツボ、漢方、薬膳など、東洋医学の各分野にわたる全15章からなり、各章は「はじめに」で概略を示し、主な英単語を1. English vocabularyに示し、英文理解の助けとしております。さらに、2. Notes **A**、**B**、**C**、**D**、3. Let's learn!、4. Additional study、5.「耳よりなはなし！」などから構成されています。

1. English vocabularyは、本文に出てきた医学や鍼灸の専門用語で、英語論文を読むのに必須の単語です。
2. Notes **A**、**B**、**C**は、本文内容の確認問題であり、またNotes **C**は、英語による出題と解答になっています。
　Notes **D**は、和文英訳問題で、本文中の英語を応用し英文を作ります。
3. Let's learn!は、本文中の重要構文や文法を説明し、練習問題があります。
4. Additional studyは、各章の東洋医学分野をさらに深めるための課題を提示しました。
　意欲を持って勉強してください。
5.「耳よりなはなし！」は、東洋医学分野での興味深い事柄を紹介しています。(p5, p22, p26, p38, p58, p65)
6.「英文法・練習問題」は、基礎的な英文法問題です。英語が苦手な方は基礎の英文法書を参考にして、練習問題に取り組んでください。

　最後に、本書を出版することが出来ましたのは医歯薬出版の皆さまのご支援によるところが大きく、心より感謝申し上げます。また、米国人の立場から様々なご助言をして頂いた鈴鹿医療科学大学のMark Laforge氏にも感謝申し上げます。

　次頁に本書の主な執筆分担を表にして示します。

2013年3月
著者一同

主な執筆分担
第1章　高木久代、木村研一
第2章　高木久代、木村研一
第3章　高木久代、木村研一
第4章　高木久代、木村研一
第5章　高木久代、木村研一
第6章　高木久代、木村研一
第7章　高木久代
第8章　高木久代、木村研一
第9章　高木久代、木村研一
第10章　高木久代、木村研一
第11章　高木久代、木村研一
第12章　高木久代、西村　甲
第13章　高木久代、西村　甲
第14章　高木久代
第15章　高木久代、高木　健
英文法・練習問題、解答　高木久代

目　　次

CHAPTER 1	東洋医学の歴史	1
	History of Oriental Medicine	
	📓 Notes	3
	▶ Let's learn!	4
	Additional study	4

CHAPTER 2	陰陽五行説	7
	Yin-Yang and the Five Elements	
	📓 Notes	8
	▶ Let's learn!	9
	Additional study	10

CHAPTER 3	五臓・六腑	11
	The Zangfu-Organs (Viscera and Bowels)	
	📓 Notes	12
	▶ Let's learn!	13
	Additional study	14

CHAPTER 4	気血津液	15
	Qi, Blood and Fluid	
	📓 Notes	16
	▶ Let's learn!	17
	Additional study	18

CHAPTER 5	経絡・経穴	19
	Meridian and Acupuncture Point	
	📓 Notes	20
	▶ Let's learn!	21
	Additional study	21

CHAPTER 6	鍼灸治療	23
	Acupuncture and Moxibustion Treatment	
	📓 Notes	24
	▶ Let's learn!	25
	Additional study	26

CHAPTER 7 治療で用いる鍼 — 27
Needles for Treatment
- Notes — 28
- ▶ Let's learn! — 29
- Additional study — 30

CHAPTER 8 肩こりの鍼治療 — 31
Acupuncture Treatment for Stiff Neck and Shoulder
- Notes — 32
- ▶ Let's learn! — 33
- Additional study — 34

CHAPTER 9 痛みに対する鍼治療 — 35
Acupuncture Treatment for Pain
- Notes — 36
- ▶ Let's learn! — 37
- Additional study — 37

CHAPTER 10 スポーツ鍼灸 — 39
Sports Acupuncture
- Notes — 40
- ▶ Let's learn! — 41
- Additional study — 42

CHAPTER 11 美容鍼灸 — 43
Cosmetic Acupuncture
- Notes — 44
- ▶ Let's learn! — 45
- Additional study — 46

CHAPTER 12 漢方薬Ⅰ — 47
Kampo Medicine Ⅰ
- Notes — 49
- ▶ Let's learn! — 50
- Additional study — 50

CHAPTER 13 漢方薬Ⅱ — 51
Kampo Medicine Ⅱ
- Notes — 53
- ▶ Let's learn! — 54
- Additional study — 54

CHAPTER 14 薬　膳 — 55
Herbal Cuisine

	📓 Notes	56
	▶ Let's learn!	57
	Additional study	58
CHAPTER 15	海外における鍼灸事情 Acupuncture Treatment in Foreign Countries	61
	📓 Notes	63
	▶ Let's learn!	64
	Additional study	64

👂耳よりなはなし！

TCMにおけるピンイン表記	5
鍼灸分野の英語表現	22
杉山和一とは？	26
経　穴	38
薬　膳	58
WHOによる鍼灸適応症	65

APPENDIX	英文法・練習問題 Grammar/Exercise	67
	受動態	67
	注意すべき受動態	68
	英文の時制　Ⅰ	69
	英文の時制　Ⅱ	70
	比　較	71
	関係代名詞	73
	分　詞	74
	不定詞	75
	助動詞	76
	解　答 Answer	77

CHAPTER 1

History of Oriental Medicine

東洋医学の歴史

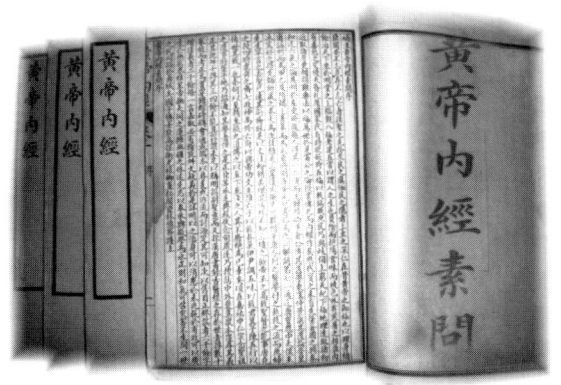 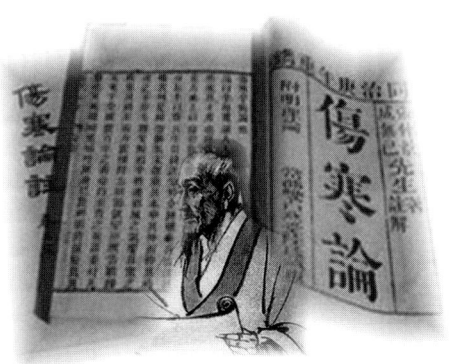

黄帝内経（左）と傷寒論（右）（写真提供：王暁明）
黄帝内経は現存する最古の中国の医学書で、漢代に編纂されました。傷寒論は漢から三国時代に張仲景によって編纂された中国医学の古典です。

はじめに

　東洋医学には漢方薬や鍼灸、按摩、マッサージなどがあります。これらの医療は古代の中国で起こり、5世紀半ばに日本に伝わり、独自に発達しました。日本では室町時代から江戸時代にかけて盛んに行われていましたが、明治時代以後は政府が西洋医学、特にドイツ医学を採用したこともあり、東洋医学は一旦、衰退しました。しかし、昭和になって西洋医学よりも副作用が少ないことや原因がはっきりしない症状や慢性病に効果があることが知られるようになって、再び鍼灸や漢方薬といった東洋医学が注目されるようになってきました。最近では医学部での授業の中にも東洋医学が科目として導入されるようになってきました。

English vocabulary

1. Huangdi Neijing　　黄帝内経（ホワンディ　ネイジン）
2. Shanghan Zabing Lun　　傷寒雑病論（シャンハン　ザービン　ルン）
3. Shennong Bencao Jing　　神農本草経（シェンノン　ベンツァオ　ジン）
4. Suwen　　素問（スーウェン）
5. Lingshu　　霊枢（リンスウ）

1. Han Dynasty　　漢時代
2. herbal　　草の、草で作った

3. abbreviate　　省略して書く、短縮する
4. doctrine　　方針、理論
5. meridian　　経絡、子午線
6. moxibustion　　灸
7. anatomy　　解剖学
8. physiology　　生理学、生理機能
9. pathology　　病理学
10. diagnosis　　診断
11. monograph　　研究論文
12. pharmacy　　調剤、薬学
13. analysis　　分析
14. therapeutic　　治療上の、健康維持に役立つ
15. pathogenesis　　病理発生、病因論
16. infection　　伝染、感染
17. accumulate　　蓄積する、ためる

History of Oriental Medicine

The oldest three books of Chinese Medicine

　　Huangdi Neijing（The Yellow Emperor's Internal Canon of Medicine）
　　Shanghan Zabing Lun（Treatise on Exogenous Febrile and Miscellaneous Diseases）
　　Shennong Bencao Jing（Shennong's Herbal Classic）

These three books were created by experiencing and practicing with some foods and their specific properties to relieve or eliminate certain diseases more than two thousand years ago. These three books became the basic theories of Chinese Medicine.

Changing of Chinese Medicine

　　Traditional Chinese Medicine（TCM）has a history going back thousands of years. The main theories of treatment have been developed and enriched by practicing throughout the Han Dynasty. Chinese Medicine reflects Han history, culture and use of natural resources.

Huangdi Neijing（The Yellow Emperor's Internal Canon of Medicine）, abbreviated to **Neijing**, is the first extensive medical classic in China. Later two more books were issued, **Suwen（Inquiring into the Origin of Life and Disease）** and **Lingshu（The Efficacious Pivot for Acupuncture）**. The former discusses the basic laws of the human body's normal and abnormal life activities. The latter explains not only the doctrine of meridians but also the essential techniques of acupuncture and moxibustion. This theory deals with anatomy, physiology, pathology of human body and the diagnosis treatments.

Shanghan Zabing Lun（Treatise on Exogenous Febrile and Miscellaneous Disease） is a masterpiece of TCM clinical medicine, which was divided into two books, **Shanghan Lun（Treatise on Exogenous**

Febrile Disease)(傷寒論) and **Jinkui Yaolue (Synopsis of Prescriptions about chronic diseases in the Golden Chamber)**(金匱要略).

<u>**Shennong Bencao Jing (Shennong's Herbal Classic)**</u> is the earliest monograph on medical herbs in China, on which the fundamental knowledge of traditional Chinese pharmacy was built.

　These three basic books established Chinese medicine's theoretical system and therapeutic principle: diagnosis and treatment based on an overall analysis of signs and symptoms. They laid down a foundation for the development of clinical medicine.
During the Jin(金), Yuan(元), Ming(明), and Qing(清) Dynasties (1200-1900 A.D.), many academic discussions took place.

　Liu Wan-Su(劉完素) stressed the pathogenesis of fire-heat and usually used cold-cool drugs and recipes. Zhang Cong-Zheng(張従正) advocated the expelling of pathogens through diaphoresis, emesis, and purgation to treat diseases. Zhu Zhen-Heng(朱震亨) expressed the viewpoint that Yang is always in excess while Yin is always deficient and emphasized the method of nourishing Yin to subdue pathogenic fire. Rich experience in treating epidemic febrile disease, including infection and noninfection, was vastly accumulated and it became one of the basic ideas of TCM.

Notes

A 英文を参考に、□内の語群より適語を選び、空所に記入してください。

　　中国医学の三大古典といわれる「①_____」、「傷寒雑病論」、「神農本草経」の3書は中国の②_____の時代（前202～後220）に成立しました。①_____は③_____と④_____という二つの書からなります。③_____には生理学・衛生学・病理学などの基礎医学が、また④_____は⑤_____に関する論文で編成されています。
「傷寒雑病論」は「傷寒論」と「金匱要略」に分けられ、「傷寒論」は腸チフスのような"傷寒"という⑥_____について論じたものであり、一方、「金匱要略」は⑦_____について論じたものであります。
「神農本草経」は⑧_____の薬効を分類した薬物書です。金、元、明、清の時代において、様々な治療法が考えられ、劉完素、張従正、朱震亨らが治療法について論じました。劉完素は熱性の病気のときは冷やす処方をし、張従正は嘔吐や下痢には病因を取り除く⑨_____をし、朱震亨は⑩_____に基づいた治療をすすめました。このように東洋医学の考え方は時代において変化しますが、この根底には3つの古典の考えが基礎となっています。

漢、生薬、鍼灸、黄帝内経、素問、霊枢、慢性疾患、瀉法、陰陽理論、急性熱病

CHAPTER 1

B 英文の内容と一致するものにはT（True）、異なるものにはF（False）を記入してください。

1. 『黄帝内経』『神農本草経』『傷寒雑病論』の3書は唐の時代に成立した。（　）
2. 『黄帝内経』の筆者は張仲景である。（　）
3. 『傷寒雑病論』では漢方薬の効能を説明している。（　）

C 次の質問に英語で答えてください。

1. When was the basic TCM theoretical system established ?
2. What is the meaning of TCM ?
3. What is Shanghan Zabing Lun ?
4. What did Liu Wan-Su stress ?
5. What did Zhu Zhen-Heng express ?

D 次の日本文を英文にしてください。

1. 「黄帝内経」は中国で一番古い医学書です。
2. 東洋医学の理論は数千年前に作られました。
3. 鍼灸師は鍼治療だけではなく、灸治療も行います。

▶ Let's learn !

━━━━━━━━━━━━━━━━━━━━━━━━━━━━━━━━━━━━━━━
Not only A But (also) B … AばかりではなくBも
━━━━━━━━━━━━━━━━━━━━━━━━━━━━━━━━━━━━━━━

● The latter explains not only the doctrine of meridian but also the essential techniques of acupuncture and moxibustion.
後のものは経絡の教義ばかりでなく、鍼灸の重要な技術をも説明します。

▶ Exercise　次の英文を日本語にしてください。

1. Not only Mary but also Tom is a good medical student.
2. I was given not only powder medicine but also pill for a cold yesterday.

━━━━━━━━━━━━━━━━━━━━━━━━━━━━━━━━━━━━━━━
Additional study：次の語句の意味を調べましょう！
━━━━━━━━━━━━━━━━━━━━━━━━━━━━━━━━━━━━━━━

1. 中国医学
2. 生理学
3. 衛生学
4. 病理学
5. 診断
6. 鍼灸
7. 漢方薬

耳よりなはなし！

TCMにおけるピンイン表記

「ピンイン」とは、中国語（漢字）の発音をアルファベットで表したものを指す。「ピンイン」を中国語で書くと「拼音」となり、発音は「pin yin」である。

中国語には、四つの声調（音の上がり、下がり）がある。たとえば、1声は「mā」、2声は「má」、3声は「mǎ」、4声は「mà」のように、アルファベットの上で声調記号を付けて高低を示す。

現在、日本で使われている漢字は中国から伝来したものが多い。漢字の読み方も特に音読みの場合は、中国語と似ているものがある。しかし声調はない。

例えば、〔日〕電話（でんわ）　〔中〕diàn huà
　　　　〔日〕多少（たしょう）　〔中〕duō shǎo
　　　　〔日〕太郎（たろう）　〔中〕tài láng
　　　　〔日〕愛好（あいこう）　〔中〕ài hào
　　　　〔日〕以来（いらい）　〔中〕yǐ lái

Traditional Chinese Medicineの内容を英文に訳す際、固有名詞、特に古代の理論を訳す場合は、2種類の訳し方がある。

①音訳。中国語の発音をそのまま表記するものである。例えば、「黄帝内経」（Huang di Nei jing）。

②意訳。漢字の意味を英訳するものである。例えば，黄帝内経（The Yellow Emperor's Internal Canon of Medicine）。

一方、Traditional Chinese Medicineの固有名詞を日本語で表記する場合、漢字（現在中国で使われる簡体字ではなく繁体字）をそのまま使用し、読み方は日本語の音読みになることが多い。「黄帝内経」は（こうていだいけい）となる。

CHAPTER 2

Yin-Yang and the Five Elements

陰陽五行説

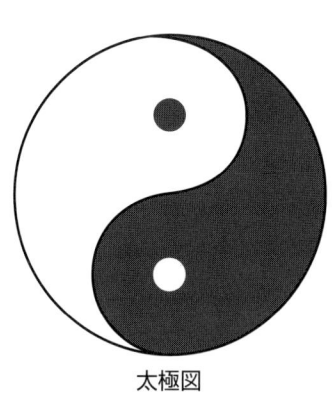

太極図

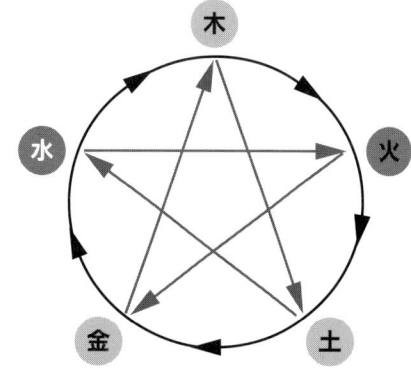

相生関係（→）と相剋関係（→）

太極図は、万物が陰と陽に分類できるという古代中国の陰陽説を意味しています。また、右図は、万物を構成する木、火、土、金、水の5つの元素には、互いを生成する相生関係と互いが対立する相剋関係があることを示しています。

はじめに

　中国医学の基礎となっているのは陰陽五行説です。陰陽五行説とは古代中国に生まれた哲学思想で、陰陽説と五行説という異なる理論を合わせたものです。陰陽説は自然界のあらゆるものを「陰」と「陽」という二つの対立するものと捉える考え方で、人体にも自然と同じく「陰」と「陽」があります。季節や時間に応じて、「陰」と「陽」は変化すると考えられています。健康な体とは「陰」でも「陽」でもなく、「陰」と「陽」のバランスがとれた状態です。一方、五行説は自然界のあらゆるものを木、火、土、金、水の5つの要素に分類する考え方であり、5つの要素は自然の営みのように互いに影響し合い、循環すると考えられています。

English vocabulary

1. proverb　　ことわざ
2. five elements　　五行
3. indispensable　　重要な
4. generation　　生成　相生
5. restriction　　制限　相剋
6. viscera　　内臓（viscusの複数）

CHAPTER 2

Yin-Yang and the Five Elements

There is a proverb in TCM that things turn into their opposites when they reach their extreme. Extreme cold may give rise to heat and extreme heat to cold. The unity of the opposites gives impetus to the occurrence, development and changes of all things, which is thought to be the core idea of the theory of Yin and Yang.

According to ancient Chinese Theory, the five elements (wood, fire, earth, metal and water) are indispensable to the daily life of mankind. They generalized and deduced the respective properties of the five substances and their relationships with each other in order to explain the material world. Among the five elements, there exist two basic relationships: generation and restriction. Generation implies production and promotion. The order of generation is as follows: wood generates fire, fire generates earth, earth generates metal, metal generates water, and water, in the end, generates wood. The relationship of the five elements in a series is all important. Moreover, the five elements generate and are generated by each other. The generation of the five elements is used to expound the interdependent relations between the five viscera.

Notes

A 英文の内容を参考に、□内の語群より適語を選び、空所に記入してください。

中医学（TCM）には、「陰極まって陽となり、陽極まって陰となる」という①_____ があります。極度の寒さにより熱が生まれ、極度の暑さにより寒さが生まれる原因となります。この②_____ が調和することで、すべてのものの発生、発達、そして変化への推進力となります。このことは陰陽論の核となる概念であると考えられています。

古代中国の理論では、人類の日常生活には5つの要素（木・火・土・金・水）が不可欠であるとされています。古代中国では、物質界を説明するために、これら5つの要素のそれぞれの特性および相互関係を一般化し、演繹しました。これら5つの要素の間には③_____ 、④_____ という二つの基本的な関係が存在しています。③_____ は、⑤_____ と⑥_____ を意味します。③_____ の順は次の通りです。木が火を生み出し、火が土を生み出し、土が金を生み出し、金が水を生み出し、最後に水が木を生み出します。5つの要素は互いを生成し、互いに生成されます。5つの要素の相生は、5つの内臓が持つ⑦_____ を解説するために用いられます。

相生、推進、ことわざ、相剋、相互依存、生成、正反対なもの

B 英文の内容と一致するものにはT、異なるものにはFを記入してください。

1. 陰陽五行説は中国医学と西洋医学の基本となっている。（　）
2. 陰陽論によると、物事は極端に陥ると反対に向かう性質がある。（　）
3. 五行の相生関係は弱いものをさらに弱めることを示している。（　）

C 次の質問に英語で答えてください。

1. What is a proverb in TCM?
2. What is the relationship of generation of five elements?

D 次の日本文を英文にしてください。

1. 金沢へ旅行したとき、たまたま私の友人に会った。（happen to ～）
2. TCMは慢性病に効果があるといわれている。（chronic disease）
3. 彼女は大学生のころ美人だったらしい。

▶ Let's learn!

時制：過去形

They <u>generalized and deduced</u> the respective properties of the five substances and their relationships

それらは5つの要素のそれぞれの特性と相互関係を一般化し、演繹しました。

<u>一般動詞には原形、過去形、過去分詞形の3つの変化があります。</u>
<u>原形の語尾に**ed**をつけて過去形、過去分詞形に変化する**規則動詞**と、不規則な活用をする不規則動詞があります。</u>

活用の紛らわしい動詞

現在形	過去形	過去分詞形
find（見つける）：	found,	found
found（設立する）：	founded,	founded
wind（巻く）：	wound,	wound
wound（傷つける）：	wounded,	wounded
lie（横になる）：	lay,	lain
lie（うそをつく）：	lied,	lied
lay（～を横たえる）：	laid,	laid

▶**Exercise** 次の日本文を英語にしてください。

1. 彼らは鍼灸師になるため陰陽五行説を勉強した。
2. トムは陰陽論で東洋医学を説明した。
3. 昨日、私は風邪で一日中ベッドで横になっていた。

CHAPTER 2

Additional study

五行説のすべての働きを調べましょう！（相生関係、相剋関係，その他の関係も含む）

CHAPTER 3

The Zangfu-Organs (Viscera and Bowels)

五臓・六腑

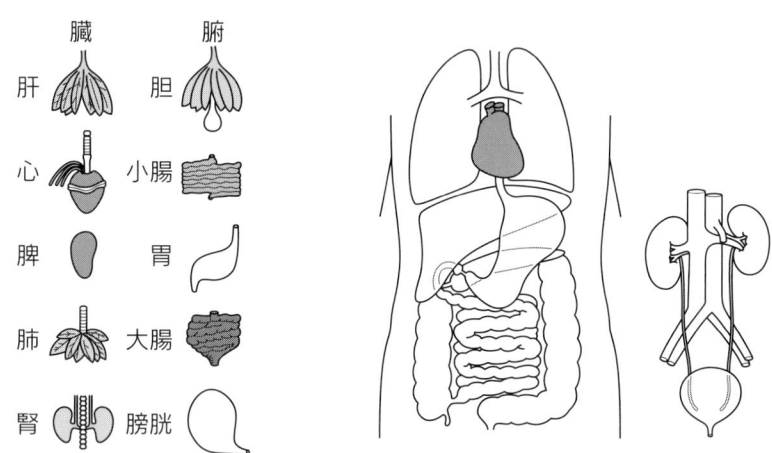

東洋医学における臓腑の形態と現代の解剖学
中国医学では人体の内臓器官を五臓・六腑と表現します。これは臓器の名前
ではなく臓器の働きを意味しています。

はじめに

　中国医学では人体の内臓器官を五臓六腑と称します。五臓は肝・心・脾・肺・腎であり、六腑とは胆・小腸・胃・大腸・膀胱・三焦を指します。これは西洋医学的な臓器の名前ではなく、臓腑の機能を意味しています。現代の解剖学では三焦に相当する臓器はありません。三焦とは水分の通路のことで上焦、中焦、下焦からなり、変調すると排尿がうまくいかなかったり、むくみが生じたりします。中国医学では五臓六腑の相互の関係を陰陽五行説に基づいて考えます。すなわち、肝と胆は木、心と小腸は火、脾と胃は土、肺と大腸は金、腎と膀胱は水というように5つの要素に分けます。これら5つの要素は相互に促進する相生関係あるいは抑制する相剋関係を持ちます。例えば木が燃えると火を生じるというのが促進的な相生関係であり、木は土に根をはって養分を吸収するので土に剋つというのが相剋関係です。このように五臓六腑は陰陽五行説に基づいて説明がなされています。

English vocabulary

1. internal　　　内部の、内面的な
2. five viscera　　　五臓
3. six bowels　　　六腑
4. extraordinary　　　異常な、並外れた

5. transmit　　送る、〜を〜に伝染させる（to/through）
6. excrete　　排泄する
7. gallbladder　　胆嚢
8. intestine　　腸、（[形] 内部の）
9. urinary　　尿の、泌尿の
10. triple energizer　　三焦
11. medulla　　骨髄
12. blood vessel　　血管
13. manifestation　　明らかになること、明示
14. anatomical　　解剖の、解剖上の
15. physiological　　生理学上の、生理的な
16. pathological　　病理学上の、病気の
17. phenomena　　現象（phenomenonの複数）

The Zangfu-Organs (Viscera and Bowels)

　The internal organs of the human body are divided into three groups："five viscera" (five organs), "six bowels" (six Fu-organs) and "extraordinary organs" (extraordinary Fu-organs). The five organs produce and store vital essence, Qi and mind. They include the heart, the liver, the spleen, the lungs and the kidneys. The Fu-organs receive and digest foodstuffs, and transmit them and excrete wastes：they contain the gallbladder, the stomach, the large intestine, the small intestine, the urinary bladder and the triple energizer. The extraordinary Fu-organs refer to the brain, the medulla, the bones, the blood vessels, the gallbladder and the uterus.

　The knowledge of visceral manifestation is based on three sources：the anatomical practices of ancient China, long time observations of physiological and pathological phenomena in daily life, and inferences made on the basis of a large collection of clinical data. The names of the viscera of the human body in TCM are very similar to those used in modern Western Medicine. Students who study TCM should understand the Zangfu-organs based on TCM theory.

Notes

A 英文の内容を参考に、□内の語群より適語を選び、空所に記入してください。

　人体の臓器は、「①_____」、「②_____」および「奇恒の腑」という3つのグループに分けられます。①_____は、生命維持に必要な「③_____」、「④_____」、および「神（精神）」の生成と貯蔵の場であり、心、肝、脾、肺、および腎が含まれます。②_____は、食物の吸収と消化、そして運搬、⑤_____、および排泄の場であり、胆、胃、大腸、小腸、膀胱、および三焦が含まれます。奇恒の腑には、脳、髄、骨、脈、胆、および女子胞（子宮）が含まれます。

臓腑論は、古代中国で行われた手術、日常の生理学的および病理学的な⑥_____の長期にわたる⑦_____、および膨大な臨床データに基づく推測、という3つの情報源に基づいています。中医学（TCM）における人体の臓器の名称は、現代西洋医学で用いられている名称と非常に類似しています。TCMを学ぶ学生は、TCM理論に基づく五臓六腑を理解していなければなりません。

精、気、拡散、観察、六腑、現象、五臓

B 英文の内容と一致するものにはT、異なるものにはFを記入してください。
1. 奇恒の腑には、脳、髄、骨、脈、胆、および女子胞（子宮）が含まれる。（　　）
2. 臓腑論は、古代中国で行われた手術のデータだけに基づき作成されている。（　　）
3. 五臓は体の臓器を示し、気の働きとは全く関係がない。（　　）

C 次の質問に英語で答えてください。
1. What do the five organs consist of?
2. What do the Fu-organs consist of?
3. What is the knowledge of visceral manifestation based on?

D 次の日本文を英文にしてください。
1. いつもは自転車で学校まで来るのですが、今日はバスで来ました。
2. バスの中はとても暑く、気分が悪くなったので、学校に着いてから、医務室に行きました。
3. 父は今夜、アメリカから成田に着く予定です。

▶ Let's learn!

時制：現在形

- They <u>include</u> the heart, the liver, the spleen, the lungs and the kidneys.
  それらは心、肝、脾、肺、腎を含みます。

1) 一般現在時制は現在の動作、状態、習慣的動作を表す。
2) 一般的事実、真理を表す。
   The sun is much bigger than the earth.
3) 未来時制の代用として使用する。
   a)「往来、発着」を表す。
   The bus arrives at five o'clock in the morning.
   b)「時」、「条件」を表す副詞節の中では未来の事を現在形で示す。
   We will start the game when the umpire comes.
   If it rains tomorrow, I will stay home all day.

CHAPTER 3

▶**Exercise** 次の英文の（　）の動詞を適切な形に変えてください。

1. My uncle always（read）a book at home.
2. I（leave）my bag in the train yesterday.
3. Let's go to the concert if you（be）free tomorrow.
4. Mary（come）back Japan from Europe tonight.
5. Five years（pass）since we（meet）each other.

Additional study

西洋医学と東洋医学の臓器について、それぞれの考え方の違いを調べましょう！

CHAPTER 4

Qi, Blood and Fluid

気血津液

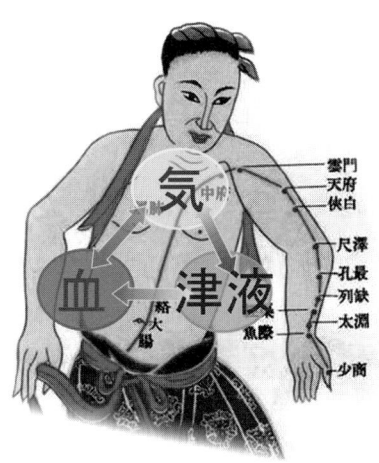

「気」、「血」「津液」の関係（写真提供：王暁明）
「気」、「血」、「津液」の三者は人体を構成し、生命活動を維持する基本物質で、
三者の間には密接な関係があるとされています。

はじめに

　気は宇宙のあらゆるものを作り出します。人体には主に原気、宗気、営気、衛気と4種類の気があり、体温の調節や血液を循環して栄養を運んだり、外から邪気を防いだりする作用があります。気が生命活動を維持しています。血は血脈の中を営気とともに循環して体中に栄養を運びます。血は心、肝、脾と関係が深く、心は脈を介して血を全身に送り出し、肝は血流を配分し、器官によって血流を調節します。脾は血の生成に関与します。血が停滞したものが瘀血です。津液とは体内の水分の総称です。さらさらした水分は津で、粘液性の水分は液で、骨や髄を潤します。

English vocabulary

1. constitute　　構成する
2. classification　　分類、区分
3. form　　構成、形成、組織物
4. inherit　　受け継ぐ、遺伝する
5. bodily fluid　　津液
6. moisten　　湿らせる
7. nourish　　栄養を与える

8. permeate　　　（液体などが）しみ渡る、浸透する
9. collateral　　　神経軸索または血管の副枝
10. metabolic　　　（新陳）代謝の
11. urination　　　排尿
12. perspiration　　　発汗
13. excretion　　　排泄（作用）

Qi, Blood and Fluid

Qi（気）is the most basic substance which constitutes the human body and preserves human life. The Qi in the human body arises in different classification and forms, and has two sources. One is the innate vital substance inherited from one's parents before birth. The other is the food essence and fresh air received from air, water, and food in the natural world.

Blood（血）is red liquid which circulates inside the blood vessels. Blood originates from two sources. One is food essence. The main source of blood comes from the food essence developed in the spleen and stomach. The other is the essence of life. Blood is from Qi, which is transformed and transported by the spleen-stomach and reddened by the functioning of the heart and lungs. It is said that Qi and blood have the same source.

Bodily fluids（津液）have four functions. Firstly, bodily fluids moisten and nourish all the organs and tissues of the body. Secondly, they can supplement the volume of blood by permeating the minute collaterals in necessity. Thirdly, they are an important part of the Yin of the body; bodily fluids are frequently used to adjust the body's Yin and Yang through different metabolic processes. Fourthly, they remove the wastes and harmful substances in the body by means of urination, perspiration and other excretion of body fluid.

Notes

A 英文の内容を参考に、□内の語群より適語を選び、空所に記入してください。

「気」は、人体を構成し、その生命を支える最も基本的な物質です。人体の気は、異なる区分と形態で生じ、2つの源を持ちます。1つは誕生前に両親から受け継ぐ「①_____」です。もう1つは自然界の空気、水、および食物から得られる「水穀の精微」と「自然界の精気」です。

「血」は、②_____内（血脈）を循環する赤い液体です。血は2つの源から生成します。1つは「水穀の精微」です。血は主に、③_____と胃で処理される水穀の精微から生成されます。もう1つは、「生命の精」です。血は、脾胃により変容・運搬（運化）された気から生成し、心と肺の作用により赤くなります。気と血は同じ起源をもつ（精血同源）と言われています。

「津液」には4つの機能があります。第1に、津液は体内のすべての臓器および組織を潤し、④_____を与えます。第2に、津液は血液の不足している微細な絡脈へと浸透していくこ

とで血を補います。第3に、津液は体の「陰」にとって重要な部分で、異なる⑤＿＿＿＿を通じて体の「陰」と「陽」の調節に大きく関与しています。第4に、津液は体内の老廃物や⑥＿＿＿＿を、排尿、⑦＿＿＿＿、そしてその他の体液の排泄という形で取り除きます。

脾、栄養、代謝過程、先天の気、血管、有害物質、発汗

B 英文の内容と一致するものにはT、異なるものにはFを記入してください。
1. 体内にある気は2つの源を持っている。（　）
2. 西洋医学と東洋医学の血の概念は同じである。（　）
3. 津液は西洋医学の体液と同じもので気の作用は考えなくてもよい。（　）

C 次の質問に英語で答えてください。
1. Explain two sources of Qi.
2. Explain four functions of bodily fluids.
3. Describe two sources of blood.

D 次の日本文を英文にしてください。
1. ジョンに昨日会ったとき、顔色がわるかったから、病気だったのかもしれない。
2. 私が入院しているとき、翠さんが子供の面倒を見てくれた。彼女にはいくら感謝してもしすぎることはない。

▶ Let's learn!

重要な助動詞の慣用表現

1) cannot help〜ing　〜せずはいられない
　　　　He could not help laughing at his attire.
2) cannot〜too または cannot〜enough　いくら〜しても〜しすぎることはない
　　　　We cannot be too careful in choosing our friends.
3) may well　〜するのはもっともだ
　　　　We may well call him a superman because he can do anything.
4) may（might）as well　〜してもよいだろう
　　　　We may as well wait for him till 5 o'clock.
5) may（might）as well〜as　〜するよりは〜するほうがまし
　　　　I might as well stay home alone as go out with him.
6) must have　過去分詞　〜だったにちがいない
　　　　Mary must have been beautiful when young.
7) used to〜　昔〜だった
　　　　There used to be a big park here.

CHAPTER 4

▶ **Exercise**　次の英文の（　　）内に適切な語句を入れてください。

1. 道路を渡るときはいくら注意してもし過ぎることはない。
   We（　　）be（　　）careful when we cross the road.
2. 今年は海外旅行に行くのをやめたほうがよさそうだ。
   You（　　）as（　　）stop going abroad this year.
3. 彼は電車に乗り遅れたに違いない。もう30分待とう。
   He（　　）（　　）missed the train. Let's wait for another 30 minutes.
4. わたしは雨の日は家に居るほうがよい。
   I（　　）（　　）（　　）stay home when it rains.
5. 以前この町には、大きな劇場がありました。
   There（　　）（　　）（　　）a big theater in this town.

Additional study

東洋医学では「気が心身両面に影響を及ぼす」といわれています。気と臓器、気と精神、気と体調との関係、気の役割などを調べましょう！

CHAPTER 5

Meridian and Acupuncture Point

経絡・経穴

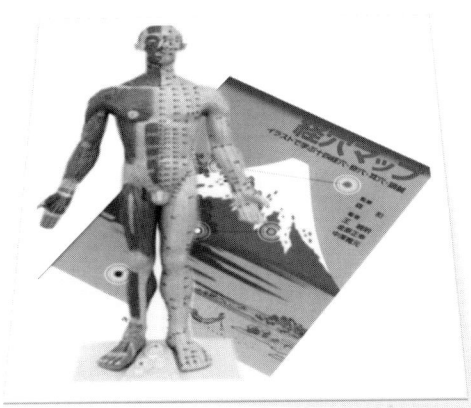

経穴人形（写真提供：王暁明）
十二の経絡と経絡上の経穴を図示した学習用の模型で、経穴人形といわれています。

はじめに

　気と血が通る通路のことを東洋医学では経絡といいます。古代中国人が身体を詳細に観察することで経絡や経穴を発見したと考えられています。経絡は臓腑に関係した名前がつけられており、12本の経脈と身体の前面の正中を通る任脈と後面の正中を通る督脈を合わせた14本から構成されています。12本の経脈はそれぞれつながっており、身体の中を循環しています。経穴は経絡上に存在し、361穴が全身に分布しています。これらの経穴を鍼灸治療では刺激し、経絡の中の気と血が動くことで臓腑の機能失調が改善すると考えられています。

English vocabulary

1. passage　　道、通路
2. Qi　　気
3. meridian　　経絡
4. Conception vessel（the Ren meridian）　　任脈
5. Govenor vessel（the Du meridian）　　督脈
6. distribute　　分布する
7. standardize　　〜を標準に合わせる、規格化する
8. stimulate　　刺激する

CHAPTER 5

Meridian and Acupuncture Point

In the concept of Oriental Medicine, the passages that blood and Qi flow through are called Channels or Meridians. Meridians are believed to constitute channels connecting the surface of the body to internal organs ,which include 12 regular meridians and two other meridians: Conception vessel (the Ren meridian) and Govenor vessel (the Du meridian). According to the theory of Chinese Medicine, when the flow of blood or Qi is blocked in one or more meridians, body disorders or pain occur. In order to improve the disorders, acupuncture helps to smooth the flow of Qi or blood through the body along the 14 major meridians.

An acupuncture point called an acu-point is located along the meridians on the surface of the body. 361 acu-points are distributed on the body and meridians have a role to connect to every acu-point. It is said that the relationship between meridians and acu-points is the same as that of railroads and stations.

The location of acu-points varied from country to country before. However the location of acu-points was standardized by WHO in 2006 after a long discussion. Stimulating meridian system including acu-points is effective for improving body condition or relieving pain of a patient.

The meridian system is thought to be located not on the surface of skin but at the place where nerves enter a muscle or at midpoint of the muscle and tissue under the skin. This is the reason why practitioners insert needles into a patient's muscle. It is a more effective treatment. But this has not been proved scientifically yet.

Notes

A 英文の内容を参考に、□内の語群より適語を選び、空所に記入してください。

身体の表面には①_____に応じて経穴（ツボ）と呼ばれる点が分布しています。この点を結んだ線が経絡です。いわば線路と駅の関係です。経絡の中には気や血が流れており、この流れが滞ると②_____になると東洋医学では考えられています。経穴の数は現在、③_____あるとされています。経穴の場所は国により異なっていましたが、WHOは④_____年に統一した場所を宣言しました。鍼を経穴に刺した際の⑤_____は皮膚でなく筋を刺激したときに生じるので、経絡は体表よりも深いところを走行していると考えられています。経穴は解剖学的に筋肉の間、⑥_____や⑦_____の分布が多いところに存在しているといわれますが、まだその実態はよく解明されていません。

臓腑、神経終末、血管、病気、361、2006、ひびき

B 英文の内容と一致するものにはT、異なるものにはFを記入してください。

1. 経絡は14本あり、経穴を結ぶ役割をしている。（　　）
2. 経穴の場所は中医学に基づいているため昔から世界で統一されていた。（　　）

3. 経絡は皮膚の下にあるという考えもあるが、まだ解明されていない。（　　）

C 次の質問に英語で答えてください。
1. How many meridians are there?
2. Explain the relationship between meridians and acu-points.
3. What causes pain or body disorders according to the theory of TCM?
4. How many acu-points are there?
5. When did WHO standardize the location of acu-points?

D 次の日本文を英文にしてください。
1. 毎日散歩をすることは健康によい。
2. 私の目標は良い治療者になることです。
3. 中国語を話すことは私には難しいですが、健は上手です。

▶ Let's learn!

動名詞

- Stimulating meridian system including acu-points is effective for improving body condition.
ツボを含む経絡を刺激することは体調を改善するには効果があります。
上記英文の下線部は動名詞で、主語の役割をしています。

動詞の原形＋〜ingの形が主語、補語、目的語などの働きをします。

主語として：Playing the piano is fun for me
補語として：My hobby is walking for one hour every day.
目的語として：My brother likes watching TV very much.

▶ **Exercise**　動名詞の用法に注意して次の文を日本語にしてください。
1. My friend's job is guiding foreign people through Japan.
2. He hates going abroad because he is afraid of traveling by plane.
3. They are good at speaking Chinese.
4. Cooking herbal cuisine is difficult for us.

Additional study

腰痛、頭痛、肩こりなどの疾患治療に適するツボについて調べましょう！

CHAPTER 5

🦻耳よりなはなし！

鍼灸分野の英語表現

鍼灸で使われる英語には一般で用いられる場合とは異なり、特殊な意味を持つものがある。

英語表現	鍼灸の特殊な意味	英語の一般的な意味
meridian	経絡（気の流れる通路）	子午線、経線
five elements	五行（木、火、土、金、水という東洋医学独自の要素）	5つの成分、要素
triple energizer	三焦	3つの元気、精力を出すもの
extraordinary organs	奇恒の腑（脳、髄、骨、脈、胆嚢、子宮を総合的に示す）	異常な器官、臓器

CHAPTER 6

Acupuncture and Moxibustion Treatment

鍼灸治療

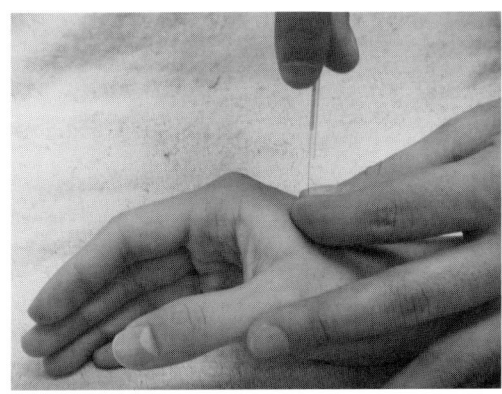 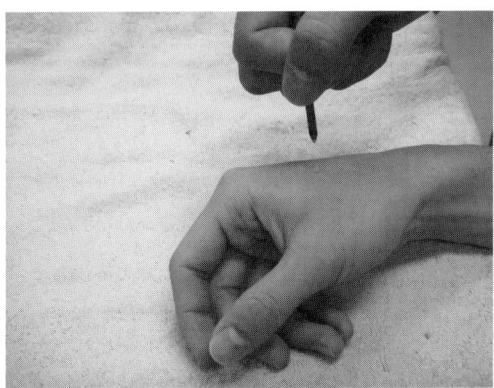

鍼治療（左）および灸治療（右）の実際
日本の鍼治療では鍼管の中に鍼を入れ、鍼の頭をたたいて鍼を刺入した後、鍼管だけを抜く管鍼法が主に用いられています。灸治療は米粒の半分ぐらいの艾（もぐさ）を経穴にすえ、線香で火をつけます。

はじめに

　鍼治療とは金属の細い鍼を用いて皮膚を接触、あるいは筋肉まで刺入し、それによって起こる様々な生体反応を用いて病気を治す方法です。灸治療はヨモギの葉から精製した艾を皮膚の上で燃焼させて、生体反応を引き起こし、病気を治療する方法です。灸治療には温熱刺激としての作用だけでなく、艾に含まれる成分に抗酸化作用や抗炎症作用などの効果もあることが知られています。一口に鍼灸治療といっても、電気治療を応用した鍼通電や、小児に対して皮膚のみを刺激する小児鍼といった方法、生姜、塩、味噌などを介して灸を行う隔物灸や棒状の灸で患部を温める棒灸、刺入した鍼の頭に艾をのせ燃焼させる灸頭鍼といった様々な治療法があります。

English vocabulary

1. practitioner　　従事者、開業医、治療者
2. moxibustion　　灸
3. moxa　　艾（もぐさ）
4. acupuncturist　　鍼灸師
5. that is to say　　つまり

CHAPTER 6

> Acupuncture and Moxibustion Treatment

Acupuncture is a treatment that a practitioner uses to cure a patient's bad condition by inserting a thin needle into the body, causing the patient's body to react. In practicing acupuncture treatment, moxibustion treatment is sometimes added. Moxibustion is a treatment that a practitioner cures illness by using moxa (natural herb), which is put on the acupuncture point on the patient's body and burned, causing a living body reaction and curing the condition by warming the body.

An acupuncturist inserts a thin needle into the patient's body, stimulating the acupuncture point and curing the patient. There are two ways of inserting a needle : Kanshinho (inserting a needle with an insertion tube) and Nenshinho (inserting a needle with twisting without an insertion tube). Nenshinho, without an insertion tube, is an original method in China and it is used in other countries except Japan. It is said that Nenshinho is more difficult than Japanese method, Kanshinho. A Japanese tycoon's acupuncturist, Waichi Sugiyama invented an insertion tube in the Edo era, and from that time Kanshinho has been common in Japan.

Moxibustion also has two methods. One is direct moxibustion called "Yukonkyu" (有痕灸). Moxa is put on a patient's skin directly and burned. After moxa is burned completely, a little scar is made on the skin by heat. The other is indirect moxibustion called "Mukonkyu" (無痕灸). Moxa is put on the skin indirectly, with something placed between the skin and moxa for the purpose of preventing a scar on the skin. That is to say, an acupuncturist puts moxa on the acupuncture point , burns it and removes it before making a scar on the skin. Furthermore, as forming moxa is difficult, acupuncturists require much training for it.

These special techniques about acupuncture and moxibustion must be mastered before treating patients. So it is necessary to study at a university or a training school where you study acupuncture and moxibustion techniques and medical knowledge for three or four years.

Notes

A 英文の内容を参考に、[ ]内の語群より適語を選び、空所に記入してください。

鍼の刺鍼法には管鍼法と撚鍼法があります。管鍼法は江戸時代に杉山和一が創始した方法で①_____を用いて行います。日本ではこの管鍼法が一般的です。一方、撚鍼法は中国古来の方法で①_____を使用せずに鍼を刺入するため、管鍼法に比べて技術的に難しいとされています。また、灸については有痕灸と無痕灸に分けることができます。有痕灸は艾を直接、皮膚において燃焼させ、皮膚に小さな②_____を残す方法で直接灸と呼ばれます。一方、無痕灸は皮膚と艾の間に介在物をおいて②_____を起こらないようにする方法です。有痕灸には③_____、焦灼灸、打膿灸があり、無痕灸には隔物灸、温筒灸、④_____、箱灸などが含まれます。一般的には八分灸といって⑤_____の上に艾を置き、⑥_____で火をつけ艾が燃え切る直前に火を消し、火傷が起こらないようにします。鍼灸

師を育成する⑦_____や大学において、このような日本独自の鍼灸の技術を学生は3年、あるいは4年かけて学びます。

鍼管、火傷、透熱灸、経穴、棒灸、線香、専門学校

B 英文の内容と一致するものにはT、異なるものにはFを記入してください。
1. 日本の鍼治療の方法は中国古来の方法に基づく。（　　）
2. 杉山和一は明治時代に、新しい鍼治療方法を開発した。（　　）
3. 管鍼法は世界で使用されている。（　　）

C 次の質問に英語で答えてください。
1. What did Waichi Sugiyama do?
2. What is the difference between Kanshinho and Nenshinho?
3. Which is more common in Japan, Kanshinho or Nenshinho?
4. How many years do they need to become an acupuncturist?
5. How do acupuncturists use moxa in treating patients?

D 次の日本文を英文にしてください。
1. 鍼灸師は火傷を防ぐためにお灸の下にびわの葉をおきます。(prevent, scar, loquat leaf)
2. 私達の腰の痛みを和らげるのはまさに鍼治療です。(It ～ that ～)

▶ Let's learn!

It is (was) ～　that (who) の強調構文

- It is acupuncture treatment that a practitioner cures a patient's bad condition by his or her living body reaction
治療者が患者の生体反応を用いて悪い箇所を治療するのがまさに鍼治療です。

この構文で文の一部を強調することができます。
that (who) の前に強調したい語句を入れ、その語句を強調する文にします。
ex) It is an acupuncturist who can treat patients with needles and moxa.
鍼や艾で患者を治療するのはまさに鍼灸師です。

▶ **Exercise**　下線の部分を強調する英文に換えてください。
1. Tom's father made this table and chair.
2. Keiko will come back from Paris tomorrow.
3. My aunt sent me a nice bag for my birthday.

CHAPTER 6

> Additional study
>
> 日本と外国の鍼治療の違いについて調べましょう！

🎧 耳よりなはなし！

> **杉山和一とは？**
>
> （？〜1694）
>
> 　江戸時代の鍼医。慶長年間（1596〜1615）に伊勢国（三重県）に生まれる。幼児のころ失明し、江戸に出て検校（けんぎょう）山瀬琢一について鍼術（しんじゅつ）を学び、さらに京都で入江豊明に師事、2家の長所とあわせ、管鍼を考案してこれを実施し名声は大いに上がった。5代将軍徳川綱吉の病気を鍼術で治療し、1692年（元禄5年）本所に宅地を与えられ、関東総検校に任ぜられた。幕命で江戸に鍼治講習所を開き、多くの門下生を養成、門下の三島安一は幕府医官となり、全国に講堂を開設して杉山流鍼術を広めた。
>
> 〔日本大百科全書（小学館）〕

CHAPTER 7

Needles for Treatment

治療で用いる鍼

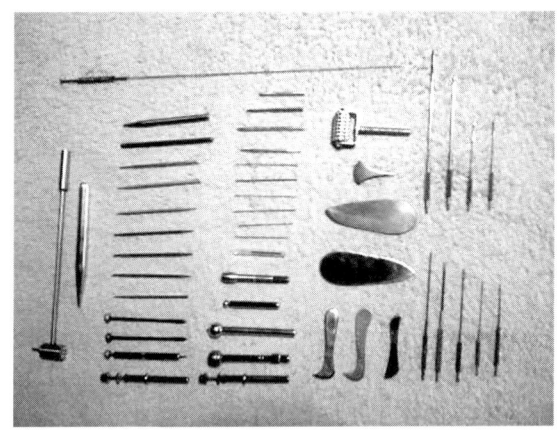

鍼のいろいろ（写真提供：和田智義）
鍼治療で用いる鍼にはたくさんの種類があります。特に小児には、痛くないように、皮下に刺入せず接触するだけのローラー鍼や三角鍼などが用いられます。

はじめに

　鍼灸治療は長い歴史があるため鍼灸治療に用いる鍼も時代とともに変化しています。石器時代には砭石と呼ばれる先のとがった石で鍼を作り、次に骨、竹、金属で作られた鍼になりました。今日では感染症予防のため使い捨て鍼（ディスポーザブル）が一般に使用されるようになっています。本章では、注射針と鍼灸治療で用いる鍼との違いを紹介します。

English vocabulary

1. Bianshi　　ビアンシ（日本語では"砭石"のことです）
2. disposable　　使い捨ての
3. hepatitis virus　　肝炎ウイルス
4. AIDS　　エイズ、後天性免疫不全症候群
5. syringe　　注射器
6. infusion　　点滴
7. pine needle　　松葉
8. bleeding　　出血
9. diameter　　直径

CHAPTER 7

Needles for Treatment

Acupuncture and moxibustion are important parts of Traditional Chinese Medicine with a long history. In the New Stone Age in China, early human beings used "Bianshi" (the earliest acupuncture instrument) to treat diseases. After the stone needles, tools made of bone, bamboo and metal were changed to the needles made of stainless or steel, which are at present the most commonly used along with disposable needles for the purpose of protecting against infections and diseases such as hepatitis virus and AIDS.

Needles for syringes in Western Medicine are hollow, so liquid can pass through. When preventing bleeding and pain, thin needles are used, while in the case of drawing blood and blood infusion, thick needles are used. The tip of the needle is cut sharply enough to insert into the skin without giving much damage to the skin.

Needles for acupuncture are not hollow, getting thinner and thinner to the point like pine needles. The thinner needles are, the less bleeding and pain is caused. Almost all of the needles for acupuncture are thinner than hair, so they are useful for cosmetic acupuncture treatment. The diameter of a needle used for acupuncture is about 0.14〜0.2mm while a syringe is 0.7〜0.9mm, which means the thickness of syringes are more than three times as thick as needles for acupuncture. The thickness of needles are different in Japan from that in China. Japanese patients prefer thinner needles because they don't want to feel pain when getting acupuncture treatment. However Chinese patients believe that feeling pain is normal in acupuncture treatment and pain is comfortable for them.

Acupuncturists need more skillful technique to use thinner needles in order that patients feel less pain.

Notes

A 英文の内容を参考に、☐内の語群より適語を選び、空所に記入してください。

鍼灸治療は長い歴史がある中国医学の重要な一部です。中国の新石器時代から、人々は病気を治療するため、先のとがった石（砭石）を使用して病気を治療していました。道具の発達は、骨や竹から作られた鍼から、金属、①＿＿＿＿で作られた鍼に変化しました。今日では②＿＿＿＿（使い捨て）の鍼が③＿＿＿＿や病気から患者を保護するためもっとも一般的に使用されています。

西洋医学用の注射は液体を注入するため、針の中が空洞になっています。痛みや出血を防ぐときは④＿＿＿＿針を、採血や輸血のときには⑤＿＿＿＿針を使用します。

鍼治療用の鍼は⑥＿＿＿＿（針状）のような形をし、空洞がないため、より細い先端になっています。鍼は細ければ細いほど組織を損傷せず痛みが少なく⑦＿＿＿＿もほとんどありません。髪の毛より細いものが多く、⑧＿＿＿＿では特に細い鍼が使用されます。鍼治療でよく使用される鍼の太さはおよそ直径0.14〜0.2mmで、採血などでよく使用される針の太さ

は 0.7 〜 0.9 mm です。鍼治療用の鍼の太さは採血用のものの $\frac{1}{3}$ 以下になります。
（鍼灸治療用は鍼とし、注射用は針と表記しました）

> ステンレス、細い、美容鍼灸、感染、太い、松葉、ディスポーザブル、出血

B 英文の内容と一致するものにはT、異なるものにはFを記入してください。

1. 鍼灸の歴史は古いが、鍼灸用の鍼の歴史はさほど古くない。（　）
2. 鍼灸用の鍼は中国と日本では同じ太さの鍼を使用する。（　）
3. 注射針は松葉のように先端が徐々に細くなっている。（　）

C 次の質問に英語で答えてください。

1. What is the difference between needles for acupuncture and needles for Western Medicine?
2. What were the oldest needles for acupuncture made of?
3. Which are thinner, needles for acupuncture or syringes?
4. Why are syringes hollow?
5. What kind of needles are used for cosmetic acupuncture treatment?

D 次の日本文を英文にしてください。

1. 今日多くのドイツの小児科医はますます鍼治療に興味を持っている。
2. トムはクラスの中の誰よりも親切です。

▶ Let's learn!

> 比較級＋比較級

ますます〜、だんだん〜

- Needles for acupuncture are not hollow, getting thinner and thinner to the point.
  鍼治療用の鍼は穴が開いていなく、先端へとだんだん細くなります。

> The 比較級＋主語＋動詞、the 比較級＋主語＋動詞

〜すればするほど〜です

- The thinner needles are, the less bleeding and pain is caused.
  鍼が細ければ細いほど、出血や痛みは少ない。

CHAPTER 7

▶**Exercise**　次の英文を日本語にしてください。

1. He is getting taller and taller.
2. Tulips become more and more beautiful in spring.
3. The sooner we begin the work, the sooner we can finish it.
4. The more we exercise, the more we can lose weight.

Additional study

　日本で使用されている鍼と、中国や他の国々で使用されている鍼の種類やそれぞれの違いを調べましょう！

CHAPTER 8

Acupuncture Treatment for Stiff Neck and Shoulder

肩こりの鍼治療

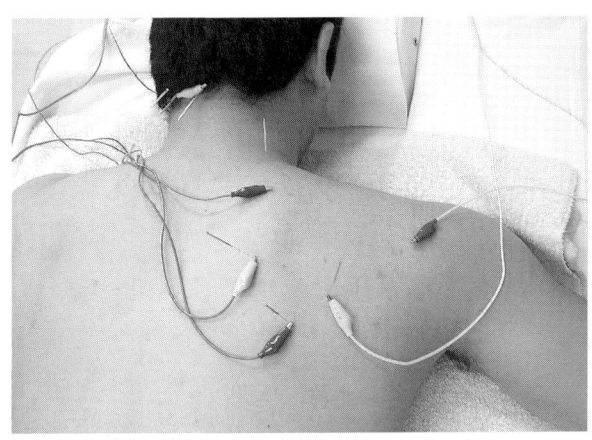

肩こりの患者への鍼通電治療
鍼通電治療とは、ステンレスの毫鍼に微弱な電流を流して
筋肉や経穴に刺激を与える治療法です。

はじめに

　肩こりはわが国では老若男女を問わず、経験する症状です。欧米ではあまり、肩こりという表現をせず、頸肩部痛の一種と捉えられています。わが国では鍼灸治療は古来、肩こりに対する治療法のひとつとして知られており、調査によると病院や診療所よりも鍼灸治療やマッサージのほうが患者の受診率が高いとされています。肩こりの原因としては運動不足や悪い姿勢による首や肩の筋疲労、精神的ストレスや夏場のクーラーなどがあります。鍼灸は深部の筋や神経の血流を良くし、精神的なストレスを緩和することで肩こりが改善すると考えられています。実際に臨床試験において肩こり患者に対する鍼灸の有効性が報告されています。

■ English vocabulary

1. stiff neck and shoulder　　肩こり
2. cervical　　首の
3. massage　　マッサージ
4. symptom　　症状
5. symptomatic　　症状に関する
6. vertebrae　　脊椎骨
7. shoulder joint　　肩関節

8. psychogenic　　心因性
9. syndrome　　症候群、兆候
10. asthenopia　　眼精疲労
11. anorexiant　　食欲抑制（薬）
12. lactic acid　　乳酸
13. potassium　　カリウム
14. metabolic product　　代謝産物

Acupuncture Treatment for Stiff Neck and Shoulder

　Stiff shoulder is the most common symptom for young and old people in Japan. In other countries it is recognized as a kind of pain in the cervical shoulder region, which is not expressed by the word "stiff shoulder". The famous Japanese writer Soseki Natume coined the Japanese word "katakori" which means stiff neck and shoulder. From that time Japanese people often use the word "katakori". Many surveys show that acupuncture and massage are very effective treatment for stiff neck and shoulder. That is why people are treated for the symptoms at an acupuncture or massage clinic more often than at hospital. There are three kinds of stiff shoulder : essential stiff shoulder, symptomatic stiff shoulder caused by disorder of cervical vertebrae and shoulder joint and psychogenic stiff shoulder.

　Recently long work at a desk and the use of computers has caused many bad symptoms which include VDT syndrome, dry eyes, asthenopia, low back pain, depression and anorexiant. Moreover, factors such as a stressful life and the use of air conditioners make the symptoms worse and the result is that lactic acid and potassium is accumulated in the muscle. By acupuncture treatment, blood flow gets better and metabolic products can be removed and so the condition of stiff neck and shoulder can be improved.

Notes

A 英文の内容を参考に、□内の語群より適語を選び、空所に記入してください。

　肩こりは器質的疾患のない本態性肩こりと、頸椎や肩関節の疾患に伴う①＿＿＿＿＿、②＿＿＿＿＿や精神的緊張による心因性肩こりの3つに分類されます。そのうち、頻度としてもっとも多いのが本態性肩こりです。最近では長時間のデスクワークや③＿＿＿＿＿の使用などにより肩こりを発症するケースが多くあります。これはコンピューターのディスプレイを長時間、見続けたことによる④＿＿＿＿＿と呼ばれる病気で、肩こりだけでなく、ドライアイや⑤＿＿＿＿＿、腰痛、抑鬱、食欲減退などの症状が含まれます。さらに精神的ストレスや⑥＿＿＿＿＿などの増悪因子によって肩こりはさらに悪化します。肩こりでは⑦＿＿＿＿＿やカリウムなどが筋肉内に蓄積されます。鍼灸治療は筋の⑧＿＿＿＿＿を改善することによってそれらの代謝産物を除去し、肩こりの症状を緩和すると考えられています。

VDT症候群、パソコン、症候性肩こり、血流、眼精疲労、エアコン、ストレス、乳酸

B 英文の内容と一致するものにはT、異なるものにはFを記入してください。

1. 肩こりは3つに分類されるが、ストレスのある生活が症状を悪化させる。（　　）
2. 肩こりでは筋肉に乳酸やカリウムが蓄積される。（　　）
3. 川端康成が「肩こり」の日本語を初めて小説で使用した。（　　）

C 次の質問に英語で答えてください。

1. Who coined the Japanese word "katakori"?
2. What factors make stiff shoulder worse?
3. What are the three kinds of stiff shoulder?

D 次の日本文を関係代名詞を使用し英文にしてください。

1. 肩こりの症状がある私の友人は毎週、鍼灸院に行きます。
2. 健君は店で一番安いコンピューターを買いました。
3. 公園で散歩している男の人は私の父です。
4. 真理子さんはいつも手伝ってくれる友人が多くいます。
5. 彼女が着ていたドレスはすばらしかった。

▶ Let's learn!

関係代名詞

● The famous Japanese writer Soseki Natume coined the Japanese word "katakori" which means stiff neck and shoulder.
有名な日本の作家である夏目漱石は首や肩がこっていることを示す「肩こり」と言う日本語を作りました。

上記英文中のwhichは関係代名詞です。関係代名詞は文と文をつなぐ接続詞と代名詞の役割があります。関係代名詞は先行詞が人のときはwho, whomのいずれかを使用し、先行詞が人以外のときにはwhichまたはthatを使用します。ただしコンマの後にはthatは使用できません。

▶ Exercise　次の英文を関係代名詞を使用して一文にしてください。

1. He cleans the new bike every day. It was given for his birthday.
2. I like my cat. Her name is MIMI.
3. The boy is the best student in the class. He is helping old people.
4. Maggie showed the pictures. She took them during the trip to Italy.
5. I learned flower arrangement from Ms. Ito. Her daughter is a famous dancer.

CHAPTER 8

Additional study

　　肩こりの症状を悪化させるVDT症候群や他の要因についてさらに調べてみましょう！
　　また肩こりに有効なツボについても調べてみましょう！

CHAPTER 9

Acupuncture Treatment for Pain

痛みに対する鍼治療

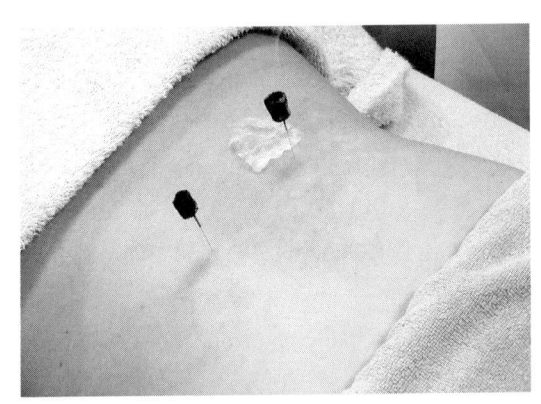

腰痛の患者への灸頭鍼（写真提供：楳田高士） 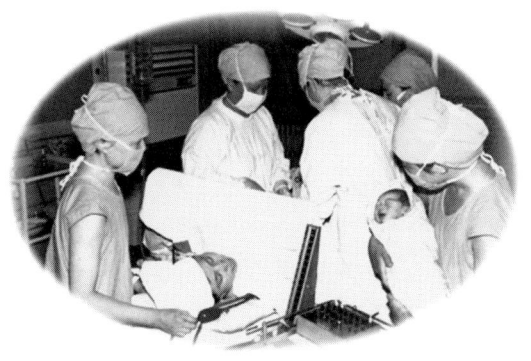　　　中国における外科手術への鍼麻酔の応用
　　　　　　　　　　　　　　　　　　　　　　　（写真提供：王暁明）

灸頭鍼とは筋肉まで刺入した鍼の柄の部分に艾をのせたもので、鍼の刺激と灸の輻射熱の両方の効果があるとされています。一方、現在では、鍼麻酔による外科手術は中国においても減っています。

はじめに

　鍼治療が痛みを緩和するということは昔からよく知られています。実際に腰痛や頭痛、膝痛、生理痛、癌性疼痛など様々な種類の痛みに対して鍼治療は応用されています。中国では数千年にわたって鍼治療が鎮痛作用を起こす手段として使用されており、外科手術の際にも鍼麻酔が試みられていました。

English vocabulary

1. menstrual pain　　生理痛
2. cancer throbbing pain　　癌性疼痛
3. anesthesia　　麻酔
4. endogenous opioid　　内因性オピオイド
5. endorphin　　エンドルフィン
6. electric current　　電流
7. naloxone　　ナロキソン
8. antagonism　　拮抗
9. experimental　　実験の
10. Zusanli（ST36）　　足三里（WHOによる表記ではST36となる）
11. adenosine　　アデノシン

12. peripheral nerve　　末梢神経
13. central nerve　　中枢神経

Acupuncture Treatment for Pain

We have known that acupuncture treatment has pain-relieving effects for a long time. In fact acupuncture is applied for curing low back pain, headache, knee pain, menstrual pain, and cancer throbbing pain. In China acupuncture has also been used as anesthesia in surgery for thousands of years. The effect of acupuncture as anesthesia is caused by applying electric current to the patient for twenty minutes. This way of controlling pain with low electric current has been studied for some time. But recently, anesthesia in Western Medicine has become the main tool in an operation in China.

The effects of acupuncture treatment for pain are composed of some mechanisms. One is related to endogenous opioids such as endorphin, which is a chemical subject in the brain that may reduce pain. One scientific fact is the effect of painkilling by electric currents is controlled by the naloxone, opioid receptor antagonism. A theory named "Gate Control Theory" demonstrates the other mechanism about painkilling caused by acupuncture treatment: thick nerves transmitting touching pressure control thin nerves transmitting pain. However this idea isn't supported today.

An experimental research with rats in 2010 showed that the function of painkilling was caused by an increase of Adenosine in the case of stimulating Zusanli (ST36) acupuncture point on experimental rats. This study made it clear that painkilling by acupuncture works on peripheral nervous system as well as on central nervous system.

Notes

A 英文の内容を参考に、□内の語群より適語を選び、空所に記入してください。

痛みに対する鍼治療の効果にはいくつかの機序があります。ひとつはエンドルフィンなどの①＿＿＿＿＿の関与です。これは鍼通電による鎮痛効果がオピオイド受容体拮抗薬である②＿＿＿＿＿によって抑制されることから鍼鎮痛の科学的根拠のひとつとして広く知られています。触圧覚を伝える太い神経の興奮が痛みを伝える細い神経の興奮を抑える③＿＿＿＿＿も古くは鍼鎮痛の機序のひとつと考えられていましたが、現在ではあまり支持されていません。2010年には麻酔ラットの経穴に鍼治療を行うと④＿＿＿＿＿が局所で増加し、鎮痛作用を引き起こすことが明らかにされました。このように鍼治療の鎮痛作用には、従来知られている内因性オピオイドなどの⑤＿＿＿＿＿鎮痛作用だけでなく、治療局所での⑥＿＿＿＿＿鎮痛作用も存在することが明らかにされてきています。

ゲートコントロール理論、アデノシン、中枢性、内因性オピオイド、末梢性、ナロキソン

B 英文の内容と一致するものにはT、異なるものにはFを記入してください。

1. 鍼の鎮痛作用は内因性オピオイドと関係がある。（　　）
2. 今日、手術時に麻酔としての鍼使用が増加している。（　　）
3. オピオイドは痛みを減らす脳内物質です。（　　）

C 次の質問に英語で答えてください。

1. How is acupuncture used in operations in China?
2. What is endorphin?
3. What did "Gate Control Theory" demonstrate?
4. Translate "Zusanli" into Japanese.
5. How long is electric current applied as anesthesia?

D 次の日本文を英文にしてください。

1. アスピリンは100年以上前から頭痛薬として使用されている。
2. 私は何度もアメリカに行ったことがありますが、アフリカには行ったことがありません。
3. 母は若い時から鍼治療を受けています。

▶ Let's learn!

現在完了の受動態

〜されています、〜されたことがあります

- In China acupuncture <u>has also been used</u> as anesthesia for surgery through thousands years.
  中国では数千年間を通して鍼治療が手術時に麻酔として使用されています。

動詞は { have been ＋ 過去分詞 / has been ＋ 過去分詞 } の形となる。

▶ **Exercise**　次の英文を現在完了の英文に書き換えてください。

1. This car is used by Ken.
2. The work was done completely by Yumi.
3. John Lennon is known all over the world.

Additional study

鍼灸による痛みに対する治療のツボを調べましょう！

CHAPTER 9

🎧 耳よりなはなし！

経穴（けいけつ）

　中国の中医学に由来し、「気と血」の通り道とされている経絡上にある。気血が出入りし、鍼・灸の刺激を与え症状の緩和をはかる効果的な場所であり、一般的にはツボとして知られている。中医学によると354穴が全身に存在するとある。WHOは1989年に361穴とした。今日、欧米では下の例のようにアルファベット2字と数字で経穴（ツボ）を表記している。

（例）

足三里：Zusanli　ST36（ST＝stomach meridian）　　胃経

三陰交：Sanyinjiao　SP6（SP＝spleen meridian）　　脾経

合谷：Hegu　LI4（LI＝large intestine meridian）　　大腸経

神門：Shenmen　HT7（HT＝heart meridian）　　心経

CHAPTER 10

Sports Acupuncture

スポーツ鍼灸

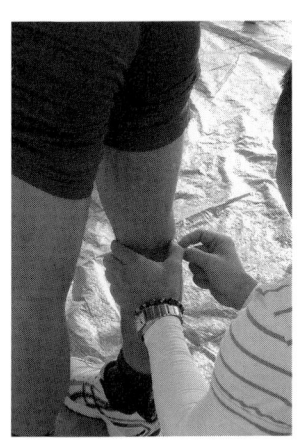

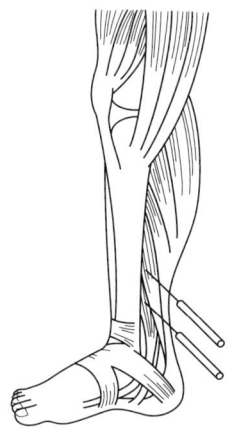

円皮鍼による治療と治療部位（写真提供：平恵一）
マラソンランナーに円皮鍼の治療を行っています。円皮鍼とは丸形の絆創膏に数ミリの鍼がついたもので、刺したままでも痛みはありません。円皮鍼を貼ったままでもスポーツが行える利点があります。

はじめに

　近年、スポーツ人口の増加に伴ってスポーツによる障害も増えています。昔からプロのアスリートに対して競技後の腰痛や膝痛に対して鍼灸治療は行われていますが、現在では一般の人を対象に競技後の症状の緩和だけでなく競技前のコンディションの維持や運動パフォーマンスの向上といった目的に対しても広く、鍼灸治療は行われています。絆創膏に小さな鍼のついた円皮鍼は競技中も貼っておくことができるので、スポーツ鍼灸の領域ではよく用いられています。実際にマラソンやトライアスロンなどの長距離走によって起こる筋肉痛を円皮鍼が軽減したことが二重盲検法を用いた臨床研究で明らかにされています。このようにスポーツ分野における鍼灸治療の効果についての研究も国内・国外で増えてきています。

English vocabulary

1. pre-competition　　競技前
2. intra-competition　　競技中
3. post-competition　　競技後
4. motor skill　　運動機能
5. fatigue　　疲労
6. muscular-skeletal system　　筋骨格系

7. muscle strain　　筋緊張
8. application　　応用、適用

Sports Acupuncture

Sports acupuncture treatment is done differently in the three phases of sports: pre-competition, intra-competition, post-competition.

The purpose is different in each phase as well.

Pre-competition

Acupuncture treatment for sports is effective for regulating athletes' body condition, which includes preventing sport disorders and improving motor skills. But acupuncture is prohibited just before competition because it makes muscle loosen.

Intra-competition

During competition, acupuncture alters athletes' experience of pain and helps them perform better, so they can do their best.

Post-competition

The purpose of acupuncture treatment for post-competition is to improve muscle fatigue and muscle soreness that occur a few days after competition. Treatment is effective by means of restoring the flow of blood in the muscular-skeletal system and so improves muscle strain.

Acupuncture held before, during and after competition is also known as preventative therapy for athletes.

Moreover it is desirable that acupuncture is combined with massage or the application of heat for the purpose of healing an athlete's body.

Notes

A 英文の内容を参考に、□内の語群より適語を選び、空所に記入してください。

　スポーツ領域の鍼灸治療には、競技前・中・後の時期に応じた目的があります。競技前にはスポーツ障害の予防や運動機能の向上などの①＿＿＿＿＿の調整を目的に行います。鍼治療を行うと、②＿＿＿＿＿が生じるので競技の直前には鍼治療は行わないほうが一般的にはよいとされています。競技中には③＿＿＿＿＿などを用いて、鎮痛作用を持続させ、良い④＿＿＿＿＿を維持することを目的とします。競技後にはスポーツによる筋疲労や⑤＿＿＿＿＿の改善を目的に鍼灸治療を行います。鍼灸には⑥＿＿＿＿＿を改善する作用や筋緊張を緩和する作用があることが知られていますので、これらの競技後の症状の改善や予防には効果があります。また、スポーツによる障害に対しては鍼灸治療以外に運動療法や⑦＿＿＿＿＿、温熱療法なども従来行われており、これらの治療法と鍼灸治療との併用が望ましいとされています。

筋弛緩、マッサージ、筋血流、遅発性筋痛、円皮鍼、コンディション、パフォーマンス

B 英文の内容と一致するものにはT、異なるものにはFを記入してください。

1. スポーツ鍼灸は試合の直前に行うのが効果的である。（　　）
2. スポーツ鍼灸はマッサージなどと一緒に行うとより効果的である。（　　）
3. スポーツ鍼灸は筋緊張を緩和するが、筋疲労には効果的ではない。（　　）

C 次の質問に英語で答えてください。

1. Explain three phases of sports acupuncture.
2. What is the effect of sports acupuncture at pre-competition?
3. Why is massage done for sports acupuncture?

D 次の日本文を英文にしてください。

1. 私の旅行の目的はいろいろなことを経験することです。
2. あの公園で犬と一緒に散歩している人は私のおじです。
3. 私の友人は鍼灸治療をしながら外国を旅しています。

▶ Let's learn!

分詞の後置修飾：現在分詞または過去分詞が前の名詞を修飾

- Acupuncture held before, during and after competition is also known as preventative therapy for athletes.
  競技の前、最中、後で行われる鍼治療は競技者のための予防療法としても知られている。

　　　◎過去分詞が名詞を修飾するときは受動態を表すことが多い。

The vase broken by the boy is expensive.
　少年によって壊された花瓶は値段が高い。
The baby crying in the bed is my little brother.
　ベッドで泣いている赤ん坊は私の弟です。

▶ **Exercise**　次の英文を日本語にしてください。

1. My father gave me a good handbag made in Italy for my birthday.
2. Tokyo Station rebuilt in 2012 is one of the most beautiful stations in the world.
3. The acupuncturist curing many patients' chronic diseases always works hard and is respected by everybody.

CHAPTER 10

| Additional study |

スポーツ鍼灸は現在，オリンピック参加競技者、サッカー、野球の選手など、多くのスポーツ選手に行われています。いろいろな事例を調べてみましょう！ また、身近でスポーツ鍼灸を行っている鍼灸師がいれば、訪問してインタビューをしてはいかがですか。

CHAPTER 11

Cosmetic Acupuncture

美容鍼灸

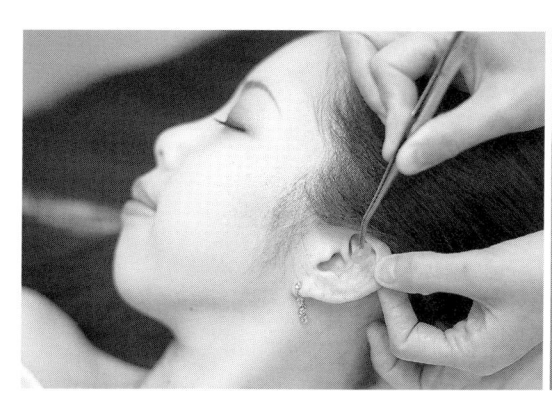

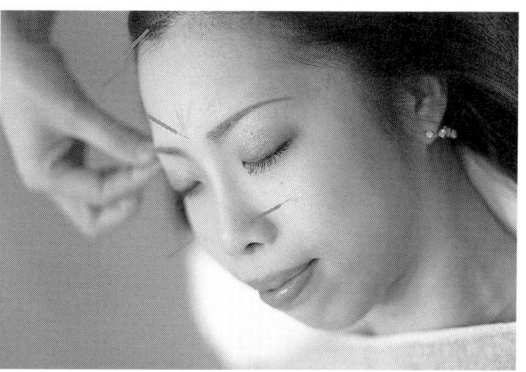

リフトアップや、しみ、たるみ改善のための鍼治療

はじめに

　ここ数年来、美容に鍼灸治療を応用した美容鍼灸が注目されています。アンチエイジングとしての美顔や痩身、脱毛症などに対して鍼灸治療が行われています。年齢からくる顔のしわやたるみ、むくみが改善したり、リフトアップによって小顔になるといった効果があるとされています。効果の機序については顔面部の血流が良くなることや筋肉が緊張するためと考えられています。美容鍼灸では顔面部に対する刺鍼が一般的に行われていますが、鍼を刺入せずに皮膚に接触する手法もあります。美容鍼灸では「美容は体の健康に基づく」という東洋医学の考えから顔面部だけの治療だけではなく、肌や筋肉の気血を補うことを目的とした治療も併せて行います。

English vocabulary

1. cosmetic acupuncture　　美容鍼灸
2. alopecia　　脱毛症
3. wrinkle　　しわ
4. bags and dark rings under the eyes　　目の下のたるみとくま
5. swelling　　むくみ
6. pigmentation　　色素沈着
7. holistic　　全身的な、ホリスティックな
8. verification　　検証、立証

CHAPTER 11

Cosmetic Acupuncture

In recent years cosmetic acupuncture has been received by many people due to its effects on anti-aging, such as making the face smaller, improving alopecia and losing weight. Common acupuncture treatment is provided to care for the patient's whole body and to cure some symptoms, while cosmetic acupuncture targets the face, improving her or his appearance: it prevents the formation of wrinkles, erases lines, and improves bags and dark rings under eyes. Moreover it can reduce facial swelling, dryness and pigmentation. A thinner needle than usual is inserted lightly at key points on the face, which causes better blood flow throughout the facial skin and muscle and improves the metabolism of the body. The theory of Oriental Medicine suggests the idea that facial wrinkle and pigmentation are caused by lung disorders and bags and dark rings under the eyes are by the weakness of the spleen and excessive drinking. An acupuncturist who studies Oriental Medicine theory always checks the patients' whole body and understand his or her body condition and way of life. Even in cosmetic acupuncture treatment, an acupuncturist treats disorders of the whole body as well as inserting a needle into the facial skin for the purpose of improving the facial appearance. This is the very idea of acupuncture treatment, that is, to provide holistic treatment. Nowadays cosmetic acupuncture is becoming common, but a verification is needed to examine its effect and safety more than before.

Notes

A 英文の内容を参考に、□内の語群より適語を選び、空所に記入してください。

鍼灸治療が特定の疾患や症状に対して行われるのに対して、美容鍼灸は顔の①_____やむくみ、②_____などの患者の③_____を改善することを目的として行われます。実際の臨床では通常の鍼より細く短い鍼を顔面部に刺入します。皮膚の④_____を良くし、代謝を改善することで治療効果が期待されます。また、東洋医学では顔の①_____やしみは⑤_____の変調によって起こり、②_____やたるみは飲食の不摂生や疲労で⑥_____が弱っているために起こると考えられています。美容鍼灸でこれらの臓腑の失調に対しても治療も行います。そのため患者の体調や生活の状況を把握することも必要です。このように唯、顔に鍼を刺すだけではなく全身の不調を整えるホリスティックな治療で美容を促進するのが美容鍼灸の特徴といえます。美容鍼灸は近年、盛んに行われていますが、一方で効果や⑦_____の検証も必要とされています。

安全性、肺、脾、目の下のくま、しわ、血流、容姿

B 英文の内容と一致するものにはT、異なるものにはFを記入してください。

1. 美容鍼灸とは顔だけに施術する方法であり体の他の部分には施術しない。(　　)
2. 東洋医学によると、しわやしみは脾の不調によるものである。(　　)

3. 東洋医学によると目の下のくまやたるみは飲食の不摂生が原因と考えられている。（　　）

C 次の質問に英語で答えてください。

1. What is the effect of cosmetic acupuncture?
2. Is cosmetic acupuncture treatment the same as the regular acupuncture treatment?
3. Why do the facial wrinkles and pigmentations occur?
4. What kind of needle is used for cosmetic acupuncture treatment?
5. Is it true that we don't need to examine cosmetic acupuncture safety due to its popularity?

D 次の日本文を英文にしてください。

1. 健とジョンは解剖学を勉強するために図書館へ行った。
2. 私は話し合える友達がたくさんいて幸せです。
3. 真理子は美容鍼灸を勉強し、将来、女性のしわを取り除きたいと思っている。

▶ Let's learn!

to　不定詞（to ＋　動詞の原形）

● A common acupuncture treatment is provided to care the patient's whole body and to cure some symptoms.
　一般の鍼治療は患者の全身ケアまたはいくつかの症状を治療するために提供される。（to不定詞の副詞用法で目的を示す）

① I need to walk everyday. 私は毎日歩くことが必要です。
② He went to the library to look for a good book. 彼はよい本を探すために図書館に行った。
①は不定詞の名詞用法、②は副詞用法で目的を示す。

▶ Exercise　次の英文の下線部に注意し日本語にしてください。
　　　　　　また不定詞の用法も示してください。

1. I went to the station to welcome the important guest.
2. Kei looked for the good clinic to have her lower back pain treated.
3. May wants to be a specialist of Oriental Medicine in the future.
4. It is important for Kei to master Oriental Medicine.

CHAPTER 11

> Additional study

今日、日本で行われている美容鍼灸の治療方法、エステと美容鍼灸との違いなどを調べてみましょう！

CHAPTER 12

Kampo Medicine I

漢方薬 I

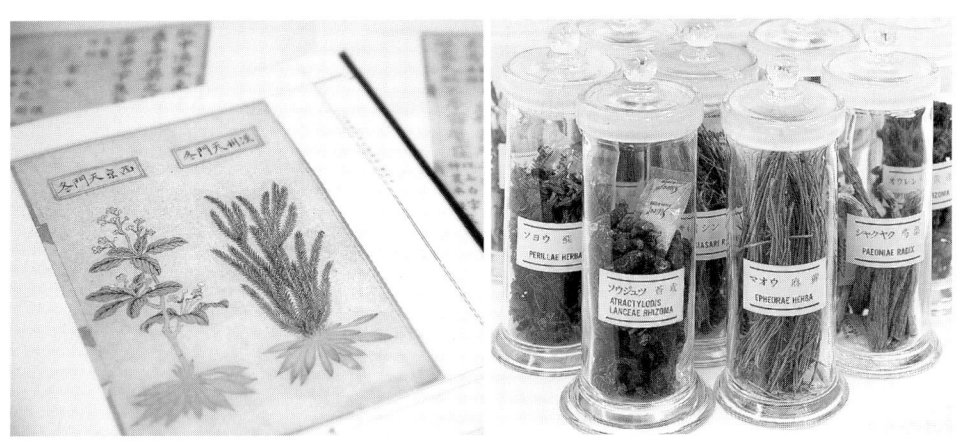

生薬に関する古典（左）と生薬標本（右）（写真提供：西村次雄）

はじめに

　漢方薬は自然の世界で作られたもの（生薬）を複数使用し、古代からの実践に基づき病気の治療、予防のために使用されています。漢方薬は、通常、複数の生薬を組み合わせて生まれたものです。生薬は薬用天然物です。おのおのの生薬には、薬味（酸・苦・甘・辛・鹹）・薬性（熱・温・涼・寒）・補瀉といった特徴があります。

　漢方の考え方には「同病異治」と「異病同治」があります。副作用の出現頻度はきわめて低いと考えられますが、予測不能な個人の特異体質もあり、副作用が出る場合もあります。

English vocabulary

1. herbal medicine　　生薬
2. Japanese envoy to Sui China　　遣隋使
3. Japanese envoy to Tang China　　遣唐使
4. dimensions　　特徴、要素
5. property　　特性、特質
6. compensate　　補正する、埋め合わせをする
7. restrain　　抑える
8. ingredient　　成分、構成要素
9. decoction　　煎じること
10. constituent　　構成要素

11. diarrhea　　　下痢
12. constitution　　体質、気質
13. prescription　　処方箋
14. idiosyncrasy　　特異体質

Kampo Medicine I

Many kinds of plants have long been used for medicine in treating and preventing diseases. In ancient China plants were used for medicine as early as 3000 B.C.. The medicine utilized with herbs in China is referred to as Traditional Chinese Medicine (TCM). On the other hand, the medicine used with herbs in Japan is referred to as Kampo Medicine. Chinese herbs are used in other countries such as in the US, Europe, Russia, but each herb is not mixed in treatment. In TCM the formula contains herbs complicatedly with no relation to ancient text, while the popular formula in ancient texts is utilized in Kampo Medicine. The original idea came from China in the Yamato and Nara eras from the hands of Japanese envoys to Sui China and to Tang China. It has been developed and completed after many studies and practices, and the basic theory which both herbal medicines depend on is mostly the same. Some ideas such as the way of combination of herbal medicine have a few differences

Kampo Medicine

Kampo Medicine is usually made from many kinds of herbs or botanicals which are made from some special natural plants and prescribed for treating and preventing illness.

Kampo Medicine whose theory is based on Oriental Medicine and the prescription is made following the theory. It has the two major dimensions. One is the temperature characteristics of the herb, which is composed of four features, namely hot, warm, cold and cool. The other is the taste property of the herb, which is composed of five, namely sour, bitter, sweet, spicy and salty. Moreover it has two important ways of treatment : to compensate for the lack of power and to restrain excessive power. Herbal Medicine with many ingredients would contain more complicated effects for diseases with decoction than we can imagine.

Though the Kampo Medicine named "keishito" (桂枝湯) and "keishikashakuyakuto" (桂枝加芍薬湯) consist of the same constituents, the former is useful for "cold", the latter with double shakuyaku (芍薬) ingredient is useful for abdominal pain and diarrhea.

Thus Kampo Medicine has very complicated effects and so it is difficult to decide which Kampo Medicine is suitable for a certain disease.

Herbal Formula

Decoction is the traditional way of preparing Kampo Medicine : you put herbs in a pot and boil them in water under a slow heat for 30 minutes or more once a day. You do this decoction several times during the day.

Two characteristics of Kampo treatment

Kampo treatment has two characteristics. They are shown with special terms. One characteristic is "treating a kind of illness by a different medicine": it is "doubyouichi"(同病異治) in Japanese, the other is "treating different illness by a kind of medicine": it is "ibyoudouchi"(異病同治) in Japanese.

For example, when treating "cold", a practitioner choose the most suitable medicine according to the patient's constitution among "maoto"(麻黄湯), "keishito"(桂枝湯), "kakkonto"(葛根湯) and "shousaikoto"(小柴胡湯). While a practitioner prescribes "hachimijiougan"(八味地黄丸) for patients such as high blood pressure, lower back pain, cataracts and urination disabilities when the patients have the same basic constitution even though they have different diseases.

Side effects

Kampo Medicine has few side effects because it is made from the safest natural herbal medicine and the remedies with Kampo Medicine have been practiced for a long time. The prescription is changed in detail by the patients' condition and constitution. However side effects such as liver disease, high blood pressure, swelling and hives are caused mainly by the patients idiosyncrasy.

Notes

A 英文の内容を参考に、□内の語群より適語を選び、空所に記入してください。

漢方薬は、通常、複数の生薬を組み合わせて生まれたものです。生薬は薬用天然物です。おのおのの生薬は、①_____（酸・苦・甘・辛・鹹）・②_____（熱・温・涼・寒）・③_____といった特徴をもっております。生薬そのものに多種の成分が含まれているうえに、その生薬を複数使うことでより多くの成分が含まれることになります。しかも、それを煎じることで化学反応が生じ、一つの成分からは想像できないような、様々な薬効を示すこともあります。漢方治療の特徴を現す用語として、同病異治と異病同治があります。例えば、感冒といっても、患者の症状に応じて麻黄湯、桂枝湯、葛根湯、④_____、麦門冬湯など、様々な漢方薬を使い分けます。これを⑤_____といっています。一方、八味地黄丸という漢方薬は患者の基本体質が同じであれば、患者の病名が高血圧、腰痛、排尿障害、⑥_____など様々であったとしても、各患者に対して適応になります。これを⑦_____といっています。

薬性、小柴胡湯、同病異治、補瀉、異病同治、薬味、白内障

B 英文の内容と一致するものにはT、異なるものにはFを記入してください。

1. 漢方薬の考えは古代から日本にあり、特に明治時代に発展した。（　）
2. 漢方薬には長年の経験があり、さらに自然の生薬を使用するため副作用はきわめて少ない。（　）
3. 漢方薬は生薬を複数使用することにより効果が増加する。（　）

CHAPTER 12

4. 漢方薬は同じ病気でも患者の体質により異なるものを使用する。（　）
5. 漢方薬は症状により種類が決められているので、一つの薬を他の症状には使用できない。（　）

C 次の質問に英語で答えてください。

1. Explain the difference between Chinese Medicine and Kampo Medicine.
2. What does the Japanese "doubyouichi" mean ?
3. What does the Japanese "ibyoudouchi" mean ?
4. Who brought the idea of herbal medicine from China ?

D 次の日本文を受動態の英文にしてください。

1. 私は風邪の治療のため漢方薬の処方をしてもらった。
2. 田中さんは誕生日に時計をプレゼントしてもらった。
3. トムは腰痛のため鍼で治療してもらっている。

▶ Let's learn!

受動態

13章の英文には受動態が多く使用されています。医療系英文では「治療される」「〜を投与される」など、受動態の英文で表現されています。

＊ Plants were used in ancient China.
　 It has been developed and completed.

▶**Exercise**　次の英文を受動態に変えてください。

1. Ken wrote a letter in Chinese.
2. They all know the person well.
3. We named our cat MIMI.
4. Yoko made a special drink for Tom.
5. The doctor gave the patient herbal medicine for a cold.

Additional study

同病異治、異病同治　について本文例以外の治療法について調べましょう！

CHAPTER 13

Kampo Medicine II

漢方薬 II

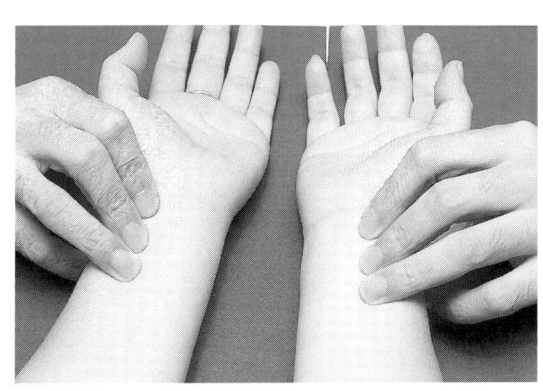

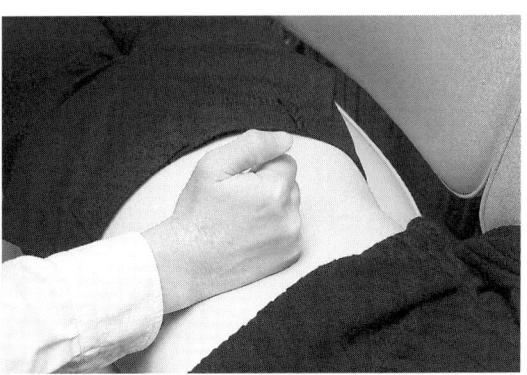

漢方医学における脈診（左）と腹診（右）（写真提供：田子芙蓉）

はじめに

　明治時代に入って日本の医学が西洋医学中心となる以前は、漢方医学がすべての疾患に対応していました。現代においても変わることはなく、疾患全般に対応しているといってよいでしょう。

　漢方医学の治療は、「本治」と「標治」からなっています。「本治」とは、体質を改善して根本から治療することで、「標治」は出現している症状を取り除いていく治療です。

　漢方治療は、どちらかといえば西洋医学の代替補完療法としての意味合いが強いように思われますが、漢方医療からみれば西洋医学が代替補完療法ということもできます。どちらの医療がより良いというのではなく、疾患の特徴や患者さんの体質などに合わせて、西洋医学・漢方医学の特性をうまく取り入れていくことが大切です。

English vocabulary

1. constitution　　体質
2. fundamentally　　根本的に
3. simultaneously　　同時に
4. characteristic　　特徴
5. hepatitis　　肝炎
6. gynecological disease　　婦人科疾患
7. generally speaking　　一般的にいえば
8. upper respiratory tract infection　　上気道炎

9. bronchitis　　気管支炎
10. pneumonia　　肺炎
11. myocardial infarction　　心筋梗塞
12. cardiovascular disease　　心疾患
13. malignant tumor　　悪性腫瘍
14. acute renal failure　　急性腎不全
15. alternative　　代替の
16. appropriate　　適切な

Kampo Medicine II

　The treatment with Kampo Medicine consists of two kinds of treatments : Honchi（本治）and Hyochi（標治）. Honchi means fundamental treatment, by which a physician improves the patient's constitution and removes a cause of illness from him or her. Hyochi means targeted treatment, which is to get rid of the patient's symptom. The two methods of treatments are often mixed or used simultaneously. It goes without saying that a practitioner often cures the patients using Honchi only.

　Considering the characteristic of Kampo Medicine and its treatment method, it has good effects on diseases such as stomach and intestine disorders, chronic hepatitis, allergic diseases, mental disorders, gynecological diseases and cold.

　Generally speaking, they say that Western Medicine is effective in treating acute diseases and some types of viral infectious disorders. However in the treatment of cold including upper respiratory tract infections, bronchitis and pneumonia, Kampo Medicine can be more effective than Western Medicine. The reason is that Kampo Medicine is prescribed keeping specific remarks such as each patient's constitution, symptoms, and the progress of disease in mind.

　While Western Medicine is more proper than Kampo Medicine in the treatment of myocardial infarction, cardiovascular diseases, high blood pressure, diabetes, malignant tumors and acute renal failure that needs emergency treatment. In the case of diabetes, it is impossible to control blood sugar with Kampo Medicine because it cannot effect insulin activity. However Kampo is useful for mild diabetes because it improves the patient's body condition by controlling blood sugar along with diet and exercise therapy. In the case of malignant tumors, Kampo and Western Medicine are used at the same time to ease side effects and improve the patients' appetite, which enables the continuation of modern anti-tumor treatment

　We cannot conclude which is more superior, Kampo or Western Medicine , but it is important to take the good qualities of Kampo and Western Medicine and treat the patient considering his or her peculiarity and condition beyond the discussion of which is appropriate or not.

Notes

A 英文の内容を参考に、☐内の語群より適語を選び、空所に記入してください。

漢方治療では、「本治」と「標治」を組み合わせ、まずは①＿＿＿＿＿で症状を改善し、次に②＿＿＿＿＿で体質を改善していく場合、あるいは2つを同時行う場合、さらに「本治」だけを行う場合があります。こうした治療法と漢方薬の特徴から、漢方治療が向いているとされるものには、③＿＿＿＿＿や慢性肝炎、アレルギー疾患、④＿＿＿＿＿、精神神経系疾患、感冒などが挙げられます。一般的に、急性期疾患やある種のウイルス感染には西洋治療が向いているとされていますが、感冒に関していえば、上気道炎であっても、こじれて⑤＿＿＿＿＿や肺炎になっても、共通に薬が処方される西洋治療よりも、症状や⑥＿＿＿＿＿、疾患の時期などの所見に合わせて薬を処方し、きめ細やかな対応ができる漢方薬のほうが、早く治るとされています。一方、向いていないとされる疾患には、心筋梗塞などの心疾患、高血圧、⑦＿＿＿＿＿、抗生物質が有効な感染症、⑧＿＿＿＿＿など緊急処置の必要性が高い疾患などがあります。ただし、これもその段階によって異なります。例えば⑨＿＿＿＿＿の場合、漢方薬にはインスリン作用が期待できないので、食後血糖値のコントロールはできません。しかし、軽い⑨＿＿＿＿＿の場合は食事・⑩＿＿＿＿＿に漢方薬を服用することで体調がよくなり、血糖が安定しているという症例があります。

> 胃腸障害、標治、婦人科疾患、悪性腫瘍、運動療法、本治、気管支炎、糖尿病、体質、急性腎不全

B 英文の内容と一致するものにはT、異なるものにはFを記入してください。

1. 漢方は常に西洋医療の代替治療と考えられている。（　　）
2. 「本治」だけで治療する場合がある。（　　）
3. 糖尿病は、漢方では血糖値コントロールができないので、軽度の糖尿病でも漢方を使用すべきではない。（　　）

C 次の質問に英語で答えてください。

1. Explain Honchi treatment and Hyochi treatment.
2. What kinds of diseases are suitable for Kampo Medicine?
3. What kinds of diseases are not suitable for Kampo Medicine?
4. Why is Kampo Medicine good for treatment of disease?
5. Is Kampo Medicine still an Alternative Medicine?

D 次の日本文を英文にしてください。

1. 東洋医学が難しいのは言うまでもない。
2. 電車に乗り遅れたことを後悔してもむだだ。（It is no use ～ ing）

CHAPTER 13

▶ Let's learn!

動名詞の慣用表現

● <u>It goes without saying that</u> a practitioner often cures the patient using the way of Honchi only.
治療者がたびたび「本治」だけで患者を治療するのは<u>言うまでもありません</u>。

上記英文の下線部は動名詞を使った慣用表現です。他に次のような慣用表現があります。
・It is no use（good）〜ing　「〜しても無駄だ」
・worth 〜ing　「〜する価値がある。〜するに値する」
・look forward to 〜ing　「〜を楽しみに待つ」
・How about 〜ing　「〜するのはどうですか？」

▶ **Exercise**　上記動名詞の慣用表現を使用した英文を4文作ってください。

1.
2.
3.
4.

Additional study

漢方治療に適する疾患、西洋医学による治療に適する疾患、または漢方治療と西洋医学治療を併用して行うべき疾患について調べましょう！

CHAPTER 14

Herbal Cuisine

薬 膳

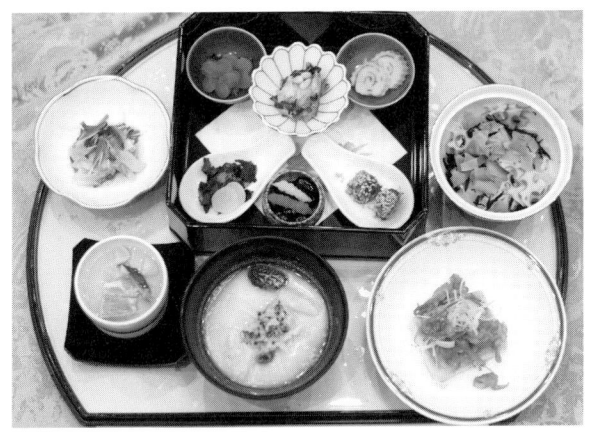

アンチエイジングのための和風薬膳料理*

はじめに

　薬膳とは中国伝統医学に基づいた食物の作用と生薬を用いた食事のことです。食材の特徴を理解し、体調（証）に合わせた食材を選んだ食事で、健康増進、健康維持、疾病の予防、治療回復の促進、老化防止を目的としています。

English vocabulary

1. herbal cuisine　　薬膳料理
2. property　　特性
3. theory　　理論
4. principle　　原理　原則
5. therapeutic　　治療できる　治癒力のある
6. constipation　　便秘
7. bowel movement　　排便
8. urinate　　排尿する
9. sub-health　　未病

---

*料理に含まれる生薬とその効能は、p59にあります。

CHAPTER 14

Herbal Cuisine

Herbal cuisine is a special dish that combines the properties of food and herbal medicine based on theories and principles in Traditional Chinese Medicine. Ancient Chinese people used some plants not only for food but also for curing diseases, which is expressed as "Yakushoku-dogen"（薬食同源）in Japanese, which means food and medicine have the same source.

Herbal cuisine consists of two original ideas: one is therapeutic foods called "Shoku-you"（食養）which means to promote and keep health, the other is the curing foods called "Shoku-ryo"（食療）, which means to make the energy of recovering illness stronger and to prevent the development of diseases.

According to the theories of TCM, it is believed that illness occurs when the balance of Yin and Yang fails. Keeping the balance in the body correctly is so important that you should choose suitable food materials in accordance with your body type and health situation, the season and the geographical environment. In addition to the basic use of herbal cuisine, it is useful for improving health condition. For example, a fig is known as a specific treatment for constipation and poor digestion as it includes much fiber, making bowel movement smooth. A squash is effective for urinating and the function of a ginger is to warm the body. Sesame is good for anti-aging. These properties of foods are also effective for preventive treatment of sub-health that is the state between health and disease. It is said that herbal cuisine is food therapy. In busier days, we consider sub-health treatment seriously so as not to develop diseases in the future. We should cook seasonal food with herbal medicine if necessary in order to spend a healthy life from now on.

Notes

A 英文の内容を参考に、□内の語群より適語を選び、空所に記入してください。

薬膳とは古代中国の①_____に基づき食物の作用と生薬を用いた食事のことです。健康増進、健康維持を目的とした②_____と疾病回復を早め病気を進行させないようにする③_____が重要とみなされていました。中医学によると、体の④_____のバランスが崩れると病気になると考えられています。薬膳はこのバランスを整えるために日々の食生活を考え、さらに摂取する人の⑤_____（証）を良く知り、効果的な食材を組み合わせ、季節にあった食材を選ぶことが重要です。⑥_____には、旬の食材を取りながら体の状態を改善する食材を加えていきます。例えば便秘や胃腸の調子が良くない人には豊富な⑦_____を含み消化を助け便通を良くする⑧_____が特効薬としてよく知られています。⑨_____には利尿作用があり、⑩_____が体を温めてくれます。"薬食同源""医食同源"の考えは食物と生薬の基は同じと言う意味があり、季節に合わせ、体調に合わせた食材をとり健康な生活を送ることを目的とした食事のことです。

食養、体の状態、いちじく、うり、生姜、中国伝統医学、食療、陰陽、未病、食物繊維

B 英文の内容と一致するものにはT、異なるものにはFを記入してください。

1. 薬膳料理は摂取する人の体調に合った食材を選ぶべきで、旬の食材を使用する必要はない。
（　　　）
2. 薬膳料理は病気の人が食する料理のことである。（　　　）
3. いちじくは利尿作用があるので、水太りの人にとって最適な食材である。（　　　）

C 次の質問に英語で答えてください。

1. What is the basic theory of herbal cuisine?
2. What are two main ideas about herbal cuisine?
3. Why is fig effective for constipation?
4. What does the unbalance of Yin and Yang cause?
5. Explain about sub-health.

D 次の日本文を英文にしてください。

1. あなたは毎朝コップ一杯の水を飲むべきです。
2. 恵子さんは美味しい薬膳料理を作ることができます。
3. TCM理論によると、なす、うりは利尿作用がある食材と考えられている。(It is thought〜)

▶ Let's learn!

> 助動詞　動詞の意味を補助する働きがある。助動詞＋動詞の原形

- We should cook seasonal food with herbal medicine if necessary in order to spend a healthy life from now on.
今後、健康的な生活を過ごすためには、必要なら生薬を入れた旬の食物を調理するべきです。

can　　〜することができる、〜かもしれない＝be able to
can not　〜のはずがない
may　　〜してもよい、〜かもしれない
must　　〜しなければならない、〜のはずです＝have to
should　〜するべきです、〜のはずです

▶ **Exercise**　助動詞に注意をして、次の英文を日本語にしてください。

1. They should exercise more for preventing obesity.
2. We must be kind to old people at any time.
3. You have to study Western Medicine as well as Oriental Medicine.
4. I wonder if my friend can be in time for the party.
5. You must not speak in a loud voice at hospital.

CHAPTER 14

Additional study

　TCM理論に基づき、健康な人を対象にした「春」「夏」「長夏」「秋」「冬」の中から2つの季節の薬膳料理のメニューを作成しましょう！

耳よりなはなし！

薬　膳

薬膳の施膳法

薬膳を作る順序：薬膳は目的を持ってつくる食事であり、次の順序で事項を考え施膳します。

主症状：人の体調

弁証：診断、症候分析

施膳方針：弁証に基づく施膳法を考える。

材料：施膳材料の選択

施膳：選択した食材で料理をつくる。（日本中医食養学会）

食材選択

　伝統中医学理論に基づく。季節（春、夏、長夏、秋、冬）の変化により、体調を整え、陰陽のバランスを保つための食材は異なってきます。特に旬の食材を使用して料理をしてください。体調が悪いときは体調改善効果のある生薬を加えてください。

春

平肝作用のある食材：セロリ、せり、金針菜

補血作用のある食材：ほうれん草、にんじん、きくらげ、黒豆、レバー

滋陰作用のある食材：小麦、えんどう豆、緑豆、きくらげ、あさり、山芋

夏

清熱作用のある食材：小豆、ハトムギ、豆腐、トマト、きゅうり、冬瓜、ハマグリ、わかめ、かに

生津作用のある食材：緑豆、キウイ、白きくらげ、豆腐、蓮、冬瓜

養心安神作用のある食材：小麦粉、はちみつ、鶏卵、百合根

長夏

健脾作用のある食材：とうもろこし、山芋、南瓜、いちじく、鴨肉

利尿、利湿作用のある食材：黒豆、緑豆、冬瓜、きゅうり、なす、えんどう豆、しじみ、

行気作用のある食材：そば、麦、キャベツ、春菊、にら、しょうが、ねぎ

秋

潤燥作用のある食材：大豆、そら豆、くわい、なし、りんご、松の実、豚肉、ピーナッツ、白魚、百合根、白ごま、ほうれん草

滋陰作用のある食材：山芋、緑豆、白きくらげ、白菜、いか、牡蠣、黒きくらげ、百合根

潤肺作用のある食材：銀杏、柿、みかん、シナモン、胡桃、松の実、白きくらげ

冬

温補、温陽作用のある食材：胡桃、ねぎ、しょうが、からし菜、にんにく、牛肉、えび、さけ

補腎作用のある食材：栗、うなぎ、海老、帆立貝、豚肉、ラム肉、卵

潤燥作用のある食材（日本の冬は乾燥するため取り入れたほうがよい）：大豆、アーモンド、ピーナッツ、百合根、オリーブオイル、ごま油、バター、卵、豚肉、きくらげ、白魚

薬膳の例：アンチエイジングのための和風薬膳料理

献立例と生薬、および効能を示す。

献立	生薬	効能
梅人参の紅花和え	紅花	血行不良による高血圧や狭心症、動脈硬化の改善
いんげんの黒ごま和え	黒ごま	皮膚の弾力を保ち、美肌効果
黒豆蜜煮	黒豆	目や髪の栄養となり皮膚を若々しく保つ
	シナモン	身体を温め冷えによる痛みを改善する
伊達巻き	はちみつ	細胞の再生能力を高め美肌や消炎効果、睡眠や疲労の改善、アンチエイジング
牡蠣のバター焼き	ラッキョウ	胃腸の調子を整え胃痙攣、下痢、痔に効果的
ほうれん草とえびの胡桃和え	胡桃	美容、脳の老化防止
	松の実	美容、アンチエイジング
牛肉の八幡巻き	白ごま	肌のツヤを保ち皮膚のカサカサを改善
鯛の酢じょうゆ和え	酢	血流改善、疲労回復
野菜の豆乳煮	なつめ	血圧の調節、免疫力向上、疲労回復
	白ごま	皮膚の弾力を保ち、美肌効果
	豆乳	美容、アンチエイジング、女性の心身をサポート
自然薯蒸し	山芋	疲労回復、滋養強壮、美容、アンチエイジング
	銀杏	咳止め、滋養強壮
豆腐ステーキの豚バラのせ	ねぎ	抗がん作用、解熱作用
蒸し寿司	緑豆	むくみ、便通の改善、美容
杏仁豆腐	杏仁	息切れ、胸の痛み、呼吸を楽にする効果
	白きくらげ	動脈硬化の改善、病後の体力回復
	百合根	咳止め、安眠
	クコの実	疲れ目、不妊、アンチエイジング、美容、免疫力向上

Acupuncture Treatment in Foreign Countries

海外における鍼灸事情

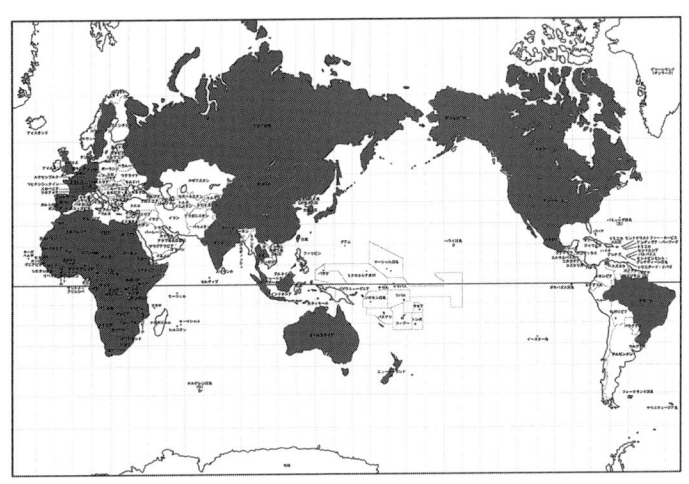

鍼灸治療が行われている世界の国々(グレーの部分)

はじめに

　アメリカ、イギリス、ドイツなどの先進国では生活習慣病など、慢性疾患の増加により医療費が高騰しています。また心身症、うつ病などの心の病が急増し西洋医学での限界から、伝統医学が導入されるようになりました。この医療は補完医療(Complementary Medicine)、または代替医療(Alternative Medicine)と呼ばれていますが、今日では西洋医学の不足を補う医療とし、補完代替医療(Complementary and Alternative Medicine:CAM)とも呼ばれています。この医療では鍼灸治療が、主要な役割を果たしています。

English vocabulary

1. health care provider　　医療従事者
2. chronic disease　　慢性疾患
3. depression　　うつ病
4. psychosomatic disease　　心身症
5. Complementary Medicine　　補完医療
6. Alternative Medicine　　代替医療
7. Complementary and Alternative Medicine　　補完代替医療
8. appendectomy　　虫垂炎除去手術
9. narcotic addiction　　麻薬中毒

10. accredited institution　　認定施設（法で認められた組織）
11. Heilpraktiker（HP）　　ハイルプラクティカー（HP）　　ドイツ独自の鍼灸師
12. midwife　　助産師

Acupuncture Treatment in Foreign Countries

According to a survey of the WHO, acupuncture treatment is suitable for 49 diseases but more diseases are cured by acupuncture treatment at a clinic or hospital. Today there are more than 160 countries and regions where doctors and acupuncturists use acupuncture to cure patients. 200,000 〜 300,000 health care providers are involved in acupuncture. Now acupuncture is entering a new stage as an international medicine.

In developed countries such as the U.S., the U.K. and Germany, the increase of chronic diseases makes medical cost higher and higher. Mental diseases such as depression and psychosomatic disease have increased so much that Western medical treatment is being restricted. And so Traditional Medicine has been introduced into clinics and hospitals. It is called "Complementary Medicine" or "Alternative Medicine". Recently the expression was changed into "Complementary and Alternative Medicine" (CAM), which means "in addition to" Western Medicine. Acupuncture is the main treatment in this medicine.

More and more practitioners use acupuncture in the U.S., Germany, the U.K., Russia and Africa. The circumstances in the U.S. and Germany are as follows.

<u>In the U.S.</u>

Americans got interested in acupuncture in 1971 when the news reported a journalist relieved his pain after an appendectomy by acupuncture treatment. It gained more attention because of its effectiveness on narcotic addiction. More and more Americans have taken advantage of acupuncture after the Office of Alternative Medicine in the National Institutes of Health was established in 1992. The method of treatment is based on Traditional Chinese Medicine. Students must study both acupuncture and Chinese herb medicine at an accredited institution to be an acupuncturist. The treatment doesn't include moxa treatment.

<u>In Germany</u>

Only doctors and Heilpraktiker (HP) can cure patients with acupuncture. But midwives are sometimes allowed to treat pregnant women with acupuncture. About 40,000 doctors practice acupuncture after training for three years. HP is German original qualification system and they have privilege of practice. Their practice method is also based on TCM. They use a needle without an inserting tube.

Notes

A 英文の内容を参考に、□内の語群より適語を選び、空所に記入してください。（同じ語を2度使ってもよい）

　　世界保健機関（WHO）の調査によると①_____疾患に対して鍼灸治療の応用が勧められ、鍼治療が行われている国、または地域はすでに②_____以上にのぼり、20万〜30万人の医療従事者が鍼治療に関わっているといわれ、鍼治療は国際化に向けた新しい発展段階へと進んでいます。

　　今日アメリカ、ドイツ、イギリス、アフリカ、ロシアなどで年々鍼治療する人が増加しています。次にアメリカ、ドイツの事情をお知らせいたします。

アメリカ

　1971年アメリカ人の記者が北京で③_____後の痛みが鍼で和らいだという記事により一気に鍼の関心が高まりました。また④_____にも鍼が有効であることに注目されるようになりました。1992年国立衛生研究所（National Institutes of Health：NIH）代替医療局（Office of Alternative Medicine：OAM）が発足して以来、アメリカでは年々鍼治療を利用する人が増えています。治療方法は、TCMに基づいています。鍼師になるためには、鍼と中国漢方の両方を学ばなければなりません。

ドイツ

　鍼治療ができるのは医師、⑤_____（HP）であり、例外として⑥_____による妊婦への鍼治療が認められています。およそ4万人の医師が鍼治療について数年間勉強した後、西洋医学と併せ鍼治療をしています。HPはドイツ特有の資格制度であり⑦_____が認められています。治療時に用いる鍼は⑧_____です。

ハイルプラクティカー、助産師、49、160、虫垂炎除去手術、鍼管無し、開業、麻薬中毒者

B 英文の内容と一致するものにはT、異なるものにはFを記入してください。

　1. WHOは49の疾患に鍼治療を勧めているが、実際の治療はもっと少ない。（　　）
　2. ドイツでは医師だけが鍼治療をすることができる。（　　）
　3. アメリカ、ドイツの鍼治療の基本はTCMである。（　　）

C 次の質問に英文で答えてください。

　1. What is an acupuncture practitioner called in Germany?
　2. What kind of needle do they use for acupuncture treatment in Germany?
　3. Explain "Complementary Medicine" or "Alternative Medicine".
　4. Why did Americans get interested in acupuncture in 1971?
　5. What do Americans study to be an acupuncturist in the U.S.?

CHAPTER 15

D 次の日本文を英語にしてください。

1. ますます多くのアメリカ人が鍼治療に興味をもっています。
2. 私達は東日本大震災が発生した日を決して忘れません。
3. あの美味しいケーキを作ったのは私の母です。（It is 〜 who 〜）

▶ Let's learn!

関係副詞

● There are more than 160 countries and regions **where** doctors and acupuncturists use acupuncture to treat patients at a clinic or hospital.
医師や鍼灸師がクリニックや病院で、患者の治療を鍼治療でする国や地域は160以上ある。
英文の波線部は前の 160 countries and regions を修飾する形容詞節です。

接続詞として関係副詞 where が使用されている。
関係副詞は関係詞の中で副詞の役割をする。

場所を示す関係副詞	where
時を示す	when
理由を示す	why
方法を示す	how

▶ Exercise　次の英文を下線部に注意して日本語にしてください。

1. He told me about the town <u>where</u> he had lived before.
2. This is the time of the year <u>when</u> you must study hard.
3. I want to know the reason <u>why</u> he got so angry.
4. This is <u>how</u> an acupuncturist treats a patient.

Additional study

世界で行われている鍼治療について調べましょう！（アフリカ、ロシア、カナダ、スウェーデンなど）鍼治療に対する保険制度、鍼灸師の教育制度なども国によって異なりますので、調べてください。

耳よりなはなし！

WHOによる鍼灸適応症

1978年、WHO（世界保健機関）は「西暦2000年までにすべての人に健康を」と宣言し、伝統医学を積極的に活用することを提案しました。

WHOが1996年に提案した鍼灸適応症のリストの一部を紹介しましょう！

運動系疾患：テニス肘、肩関節周囲炎、慢性関節リウマチ、捻挫と打撲

消化器・呼吸器系疾患：下痢、便秘、潰瘍性腸症候群、急性へんとう炎、咽頭炎

疼痛疾患：頭痛、片頭痛、坐骨神経痛、ヘルペス後神経痛

循環器系疾患：狭心症を伴う虚血性心疾患、高血圧症、低血圧症、不整脈

泌尿・産婦人科系疾患：月経困難症、月経異常、女性不妊、尿失禁

その他の疾患：近視、肥満、メニエール症候群、うつ病、薬物中毒

APPENDIX

Grammar/Exercise

英文法・練習問題

受動態

The bread was cut by Mary with a knife.（受動態、動作を受けるものが主語になる。～される）
Mary cut the bread with a knife.（能動態　動作するものが主語になる。～する）
1) 受動態の動詞は be動詞＋過去分詞 で表される。

受動態の時制

My shirt is washed every day.（現在形）
　　　　 will be washed every day.（未来形）
　　　　 has been washed every day.（現在完了形）
　　　　 must be washed every day.（助動詞とともに）
　　　　 is being washed every day.（進行形とともに）

2) 能動態の目的語が受動態の主語になる。
3) 能動態の主語を受動態では行為者として表す。 by～として示す。

　　＊感情、心理は by 以外の前置詞で表される。

be absorbed in	～に熱中している
be disappointed at	～に失望する
be pleased with	～に喜ぶ
be satisfied with	～に満足する
be interested in	～に興味を持つ
be worried about	～を心配する
be frightened of	～におびえる

▶ Exercise

A 次の英文を受動態に変えてください。また受動態の英文は平叙文に変えてください。

1. I have not finished my work yet.
2. We must keep this room clean all the time
3. They all know the person well.
4. Oates could not keep up with his companions.
5. Are they solving that difficult problem now ?

6. My father will buy a new computer tomorrow.

7. They are carrying the injured to the hospital.

8. We named our cat MIMI.

9. Who built that beautiful house?

10. The patient was given much medicine to get well at the hospital

B 次の英文の空欄に適切な前置詞を入れてください．

1. The mountains are covered (　　) snow.

2. The women were dressed (　　) red.

3. The tent was made (　　) waterproof cloth.

4. My father was very satisfied (　　) my grade

5. Many passengers were injured (　　) the accident.

6. People in the country make special rice (　　) special sake.

7. The bus was filled (　　) people.

8. His son was killed (　　) World War Ⅱ.

9. They were acquainted (　　) each other.

10. Wine is made (　　) grapes.

C 次の日本文を英文にしてください。

1. 私の弟は、自動車にはねられたので、すぐ病院に運ばれた。

2. 彼は入院しているとき、看護師さんによく世話をしてもらった。

3. 私は誕生日に父から贈られた、ネックレスに大変満足しています

注意すべき受動態

感情、被害を表すものは、日本語では受身にならないが英語では受動態で能動態の意味を表す。

be surprised at	be injured	be frightened of	
be satisfied with	be wounded		
be pleased with	be worried about		
be disappointed at	be shocked at		
be absorbed in	「～に熱中している」	be tired of	「～に飽きている」
be convinced of	「～を確信している」	be accustomed to	「～に慣れている」

群動詞の受動態…群動詞はひとまとまりと考え、受動態にするときは動詞だけを変化させる。

Nurses take care of many patients in hospital.

Many patients are taken care of by nurses in hospital.

群動詞

look after　　speak of　　put off　　bring up
look up to「〜を尊敬する」　　catch up with「〜に追いつく」　　lose sight of「〜を見失う」
make fun of「〜をからかう」　　do away with「〜を廃止する」　　put up with「〜を我慢する」
put an end to「〜を終わりにする」　　make little of「〜を軽んじる」

▶Exercise

A 次の英文を受動態に変えてください。
1. Someone saw him take the purse.
2. I will have John repair my chair.
3. We made the dog sit quietly before eating.
4. I couldn't catch up with Tom.
5. Students always speak well of that teacher.

B 次の日本文を英文にしてください。
1.「ロミオとジュリエット」は誰にでも知られているシェークスピアの悲劇です。
2. 私は昨日京都駅で、ウール製のかわいい帽子を買った。

英文の時制　Ⅰ

一般現在
1) 一般現在時制は現在の動作、状態、習慣的動作を表す。
2) 一般的事実、真理を表す。
　　The sun is much bigger than the earth.
3) 未来時制の代用として使用する。
　a)「往来、発着」を表す。
　　The bus arrives at seven o'clock every morning.
　b)「時」、「条件」を表す副詞節の中で。
　　We will start the game when the umpire comes.
　　If it rains tomorrow, I will stay home all day.

現在完了
1) 現在までの動作の完了を表す。（もう〜してしまった）
　　I have already finished my homework.
2) 過去の動作が現在に影響を及ぼしている。
　　My father has given up smoking recently.（He doesn't smoke now.）
3) 現在までの経験を表す。（〜したことがある）
　　Have you ever been to Paris？

＊明確な日時を表す語句（yesterday, ～ago, last year, when）を用いるときは過去形を使用する。完了形は使用できない。

▶ Exercise

A 次の英文の（　）の動詞を適切な形に変えてください。

1. My uncle（read）a book when I visited his house.
2. I（lose）my purse while I（see）the sights of the city.
3. If you（be）free tomorrow, I will take you to the museum.
4. I（clean）my room since this morning because many guests will come to my house.
5. Ten years（pass）since we（leave）my home.
6. I think Mary（travel）in England at this time next spring.
7. Five times six（be）thirty.
8. My mother（know）Mr. White for thirty years.
9. His cousin（be）ill in bed for a week when I called him.
10. I want to know when Mary（visit）Japan if you（hear）from her.

B 次の日本文を英文にしてください。

1. 私が言ったように勉強したら、あなたの英語能力が伸びるのは確かだと思います。

英文の時制　Ⅱ

過去完了

1) 過去のあるときまでの動作の完了を表す。「～してしまっていた」

When I entered the room, the teacher had already started the class.

2) 過去のある時までの経験を表す。「～したことがあった」

Tom borrowed the video, but he had seen it before.

▶ Exercise

A 次の英文を日本語にしてください。

1. They will have been building the bridge for six years next month.
2. He had known her for ten years when they got married.
3. Have you ever thought that you might be mistaken?
4. She couldn't help getting angry when they laughed at her.
5. I wonder when he will come back to Japan.

B 次の日本文を英文にしてください。
1. 今出かければ、12時の「のぞみ」に間に合いますよ。
2. 私はまだ富士山に登ったことがないので、今年の夏に登る予定です。
3. 私の弟は去年アメリカから日本に帰ってきました。彼は15年もアメリカで薬剤師をしていたので、去年一年は日本のシステムに慣れるのに苦労したようです。

比　較

比較…比較変化、原級による比較、比較級による比較、最上級による比較

比較変化…不規則変化の例

good（よい） well（よく）	better better	best best	old（年をとった）		older elder	oldest eldest（年上の）
bad（悪い） ill（病気の）	worse worse	worst worst	far（遠い）	距離を示す 程度を示す	farther further	farthest furthest（さらに）
many（多数の） much（多量の）	more more	most most	late（遅い）	時間を示す 順番を示す	later latter（あと）	latest last（さいご）
little（少量の）	less	least				

原級による比較

　　My father is as old as your father.

　　John is not so tall as Tom.

　　My house is twice as large as Mary's.

比較級による比較

　　The patient feels better today than yesterday.

　　Tokyo is much larger than Suzuka.

　　Sue is the taller of the two.

最上級による比較

　　I like spring (the) best in the year.

　　Your idea is by far the best of all.

　　I am happiest when I cook.

比較の慣用表現

1. You should read as many books as you can when you are young. (as ～ as possible)

　　「できるだけ～」as ～ as one can

2. Shakespeare is not so much a poet as a dramatist.

　　not so much A as B「AというよりはむしろB」= B rather than A

3. The higher we climb the mountain, the cooler it becomes.

　　The ＋比較級、The ＋比較級 =「～すればするほど（ますます）…」

4. The boys in my class are getting taller and taller.

　　比較級＋比較級 =「ますます～」

5. We must make the most of our opportunity at school.

APPENDIX

make the most（best）of ＝「最大限に利用する」

6. He is the last person to tell a lie.

　　The last…to do 〜「最も〜しそうにない」

7. A whale is no more a fish than a horse is.

　　no more 〜 than B「〜でないのはBと同じである」「Bと同様〜でない」

8. A whale is no less a mammal than a horse is.

　　no less 〜 than B「〜であるのはBと同じである」「Bと同様〜である」

9. I could get no more than two thousand yen in spite of having worked all day.

　　no more than ＝ only

10. He spent no less than one million yen for his trip to Europe.

　　no less than ＝ as many（much）as

▶Exercise

A 次の英文の空欄に適切な語句を入れてください。

1. 彼女はあいかわらず綺麗だね。

　　She is（　）beautiful（　）（　）, isn't she ?

2. 健康ほど大切なものはない。

　　Nothing is（　）（　）than health.

3. 1ヵ月に1万円しか使わなかった。

　　I spent（　）（　）（　）10,000 yen a month.

4. 彼は100万ドルも貯めた。

　　He could save（　）（　）（　）one million dollars.

5. 欠点があるからなおさら彼女のことが好き。

　　I love her all（　）（　）for her faults.

6. あなたはそんなばかげたことを言うほどばかではない。

　　You should know（　）（　）（　）say the folly things .

7. この酒はあの酒よりいい。

　　This Sake is（　）to that one.

8. 昨夜は暖かいというより暑かった。

　　It was not（　）（　）warm（　）hot last night.

9. 私達はできる限り一生懸命働くべきだ。

　　We must work（　）hard（　）we（　）

10. 私達は今年与えられた機会を十分使うべきです。

　　We should make（　）（　）（　）our opportunity this year.

B 次の日本文を英文にしてください。

1. 彼女は少なくとも日本に3人、アメリカに2人の仲のよい友人がいます。

関係代名詞

関係代名詞…接続詞と代名詞の働きをし、形容詞節を導く。

関係代名詞には who, whose, whom, which, that, what がある。

・who…先行詞が人で、主格の場合。

I have a friend who can speak English well.

・whom…先行詞が人で、目的格の場合。（省略できる）

Tom is a good boy whom every teacher praises.

・which…先行詞が物、動物で、主格と目的格の場合。

I know that building which is the oldest in Japan.

This is the chair which my father made last year.

・that…先行詞の種類に関係なく、主格と目的格の場合。先行詞に形容詞の最上級、all, the only, no などがついた場合。

He is the best student that studies French in this class.

・whose…先行詞が人、物、動物で所有格の場合。

I have a friend whose father is a famous pianist.

・what…先行詞を含む関係代名詞。

Please tell what you think. what = the thing which

・what を含む慣用表現。

what is called いわゆる　　what is better（worse）さらによいことには（悪いことには）

what is more さらに　　what ～ used to be（is, are, was, were）以前の～、今の～

▶ Exercise

A 次の英文の空欄に適切な関係代名詞を入れてください。

1. There were many children （　　） parents were killed in the war.
2. Tom is different from （　　） he was in youth.
3. This is the book （　　） my uncle gave me when I entered elementary school.
4. Bob bought a new car, （　　） he is very proud of.
5. Have you ever visited the place in （　　） Shakespeare was born.
6. My mother made me （　　） I am today.
7. Look at the woman and the dog （　　） are walking along the street.
8. The lady （　　） we met at the station is Tom's mother.
9. I am sure （　　） Jane said yesterday was a lie.
10. She is the only girl （　　） can solve this problem in this class.

B 次の日本文を英文にしてください。

1. 彼は今朝バスに乗り遅れ、さらに悪いことに宿題を家に忘れた。

2. 彼の大好きなことは、友人と海外旅行することです。

3. 朝ご飯を食べない子供は授業中に集中力に欠けるようです。

分　詞

分詞　1. 分詞の限定用法

　　　2. 分詞の叙述用法（主格補語、目的格補語）

1. 分詞の限定用法…分詞が名詞を修飾する。（分詞の形容詞用法）

　　　現在分詞（〜ing）：「〜している、〜する」の意味で名詞を修飾する。

　　　過去分詞：「〜される、〜された」の意味で名詞を修飾する。

・Look at the crying baby.（分詞だけのときは名詞の前に置く）

　Look at the baby crying in the bed.（分詞が他の語句を伴うときは名詞の後におく）

・I found the hidden treasure.

　I found the treasure hidden in the cave.

2. 分詞の述語用法…分詞が補語の働きをする。

・主格補語としての働きをする。

　The bird came flying through the window.（〜しながら）

　The teacher sat surrounded by many students.（〜されて）

・目的格補語としての働きをする。

　I saw the boy playing soccer in the park.

　Mary heard her name called at the department store yesterday.

▶Exercise

A 次の英文の（　）内の動詞を適切な形に変えてください。

1. When did you have your car（repair）?
2. He spent a lot of money（travel）around the world.
3. My friend has many bags（make）in France.
4. He left the class（satisfy）with his result of the test.
5. English is the language（speak）in many countries.
6. The student（study）hard in the library is my brother.
7. The（injure）were being carried to hospital.
8. The old man（read）a book under the tree seemed to enjoy his life.
9. He was pleased to make himself（understand）at the meeting.
10. Do you know the woman（wait）for the bus over there?

B 次の日本文を英文にしてください。

1. 私はスーザンが公園で日光浴をしているのを見ました。

2. 彼女はイタリアで日本製のかばんを買ってしまった。

3. 川で魚釣りをしているあの男の人は私の叔父です。今晩叔父から生きのいい魚が我が家に届くことを期待しています。

不定詞

1) 形容詞＋to動詞　ある形容詞は不定詞を受ける。

I am happy to meet you again.

He was very sorry to have kept me waiting.

His companions were eager to battle for their country.

2) too＋形容詞／形容詞＋enough／so＋形容詞＋to動詞

あまりにも〜過ぎて〜できない、〜するほど（十分）〜だ

He was too tired to walk any more.

The ice is thick enough for us to skate on.

He is so kind as to help me do my homework.

3) to＋動詞は副詞的にも用いられ、目的、理由、原因、結果を表す。

（目的）〜するために

We left home early in order to catch the first train this morning.

He must study hard to pass the examination.

（結果）結果〜だ

He grew up to be a great scientist.

I woke to find myself in the hospital.

（理由）〜とは

He must be a gentleman to repair the broken chair for the old lady.

▶ Exercise

A 次の英文を日本語にしてください。

1. This book is too difficult for me to read.

2. He is not rich enough to buy a house with a fine garden.

3. We ran fast in order to catch the last bus.

B 次の日本文を英文にしてください。

1. 昨日私は、偶然トムと同じ電車に乗りました。

2. あの数学の問題は難しすぎて、私は解くことができなかった。

助動詞

助動詞：動詞（本動詞）の前について動詞を手助けするものである。

1) can：可能、許可、依頼、可能性の推量

　　I can swim well.

　　You can eat this cake.

　　Can you help me with my homework？

　　That boy cannot be generous to say such an impolite thing.

2) may：許可、可能性の推量

　　May I go home？　No, you may not.（must not）

　　It may rain tonight.

3) must：義務、断定的推量

　　You must return the book when you have finished reading it.

　　He must be an American judging from his English pronunciation.

4) should：義務、当然

　　You should be quiet so as not to wake the baby.

　　This dictionary should help you very much.

5) 過去のことに対する推量

　　cannot have ＋過去分詞〜したはずがない

　　may have ＋過去分詞〜したかもしれない

　　must have ＋過去分詞〜したに違いない

　　should have ＋過去分詞〜すべきだったの

▶Exercise

A 次の英文の空欄に適切な助動詞を入れてください。

1.（　　）I start now？　No, you don't have to start now.

2. He is running along the river now. He（　　）be ill.

3. It is natural that they（　　）take care of their parents.

4. Tom（　　）not let John enter the room yesterday.

5. He runs very fast. He（　　）be still young.

B 次の日本文を英文にしてください。

1. 彼が君の意見に賛成するとは驚きだ。

2. メアリーのお母さんは若いころ美人だったに違いない。

ANSWER

解 答

CHAPTER 1　History of Oriental Medicine
東洋医学の歴史

NOTES　p3

A　① 黄帝内経　② 漢　③ 素問　④ 霊枢　⑤ 鍼灸　⑥ 急性熱病　⑦ 慢性疾患　⑧ 生薬　⑨ 瀉法　⑩ 陰陽理論

B　1. F　2. F　3. F

C　1. It was established more than two thousand years ago.
2. It means Traditional Chinese Medicine.
3. It is a masterpiece of TCM clinical medicine.
4. He stressed the pathogenesis of fire-heat and used cold-cool drugs and recipes.
5. He expressed the viewpoint that Yang is always in excess while Yin is deficient.

D　1. "Huangdi Neijing" is the oldest medical book in China.
2. The theory of Oriental Medicine was established thousands years ago.
3. Not only acupuncture but also moxibustion are used for treatment by an acupuncturist.

▶ Let's learn!　p4

▶ Exercise

1. メアリーばかりではなくトムもよい医学生です。
2. 私は昨日風邪のために粉薬だけではなく錠剤ももらいました。

CHAPTER 2　Yin-Yang and the Five Elements
陰陽五行説

NOTES　p8

A　① ことわざ　② 正反対なもの　③ 相生　④ 相剋　⑤ 生成　⑥ 推進　⑦ 相互依存

B　1. F　2. T　3. F

C　1. It is that things turn into their opposites when they reach their extreme.
2. It is that generation implies production and promotion.

D　1. I happened to meet a friend of mine during the trip to Kanazawa.
2. They say that TCM is effective against chronic diseases.
　　TCM is said to be effective against chronic diseases.
3. They say that she was beautiful when she was a college student.

APPENDIX

▶ Let's learn!　p9

　▶Exercise

　1. They studied the theory of Yin-Yang and Five Elements to be an acupuncturist.
　2. Tom explained Oriental Medicine with Yin-Yang theory.
　3. Yesterday, I was in bed all day with a cold.

CHAPTER 3　The Zangfu-Organs（Viscera and Bowels）
五臓・六腑

■ Notes　p12

A ① 五臓　② 六腑　③ 気　④ 精　⑤ 拡散　⑥ 現象　⑦ 観察

B 1. T　2. F　3. F

C 1. They consist of the heart, the liver, the spleen, the lungs and the kidneys.
　　2. They consist of the gallbladder, the stomach, the large intestine, the small intestine, the urinary bladder and the triple energizer.
　　3. It is based on the anatomical practices of ancient China, long time observations of physiological and pathological phenomena in daily life, and inferences made on the basis of a large collection of clinical data.

D 1. I usually come to school by bicycle, but today I came by bus.
　　2. In the bus it was very hot and so I felt ill. I went to the medical room after arriving at school.
　　3. My father is arriving at Narita from America tonight.

▶ Let's learn!　p13

　▶Exercise

　1. reads　2. left　3. are　4. will come または, is coming　5. have passed, met

CHAPTER 4　Qi, Blood and Fluid
気血津液

■ Notes　p16

A ① 先天の気　② 血管　③ 脾　④ 栄養　⑤ 代謝過程　⑥ 有害物質　⑦ 発汗

B 1. T　2. F　3. F

C 1. One is the innate vital substance inherited from one's parents before birth, the other is the food essence and fresh air received from air, water, and food in the natural world.
　　2. 1. To moisten and nourish all the organs and tissues. 2. To supply the volume of blood.
　　　3. To play an important part of the Yin of the body.
　　　4. To remove the wastes and harmful substances in the body.
　　3. One is food essence and the other is the essence of life.

D 1. John may have been sick because he looked pale when I met him yesterday.

2. Midori took care of my children when I was in the hospital. I cannot appreciate her too much.

▶ Let's learn!   p17

▶ Exercise

1. cannot, too   2. may, well   3. must, have   4. may, as, well   5. used, to, be

CHAPTER 5　Meridian and Acupuncture Point
経絡・経穴

■ NOTES   p20

A ① 臓腑　② 病気　③ 361　④ 2006　⑤ ひびき　⑥⑦ 血管、神経終末（順不同）

B 1. T   2. F   3. T

C 1. There are 14 meridians：12 regular meridians and two other meridians.

2. The relation between them is the same as that of railroads and stations.

3. The blocking of the flow of blood and Qi does.

4. There are 361 acu-points.

5. WHO did it in 2006.

D 1. It is healthy to walk every day.

　Walking every day is good for health.

2. My aim is to be a good practitioner.

3. It is difficult for me to speak Chinese, but Ken is good at speaking Chinese.

▶ Let's learn!   p21

▶ Exercise

1. 私の友人の仕事は、外国人を日本中案内することです。

2. 彼は飛行機で旅行することが怖いので、外国に行くことが大嫌いです。

3. 彼らは中国語を話すことが上手です。

4. 薬膳を調理することは私たちにとって難しい。

CHAPTER 6　Acupuncture and Moxibustion Treatment
鍼灸治療

■ NOTES   p24

A ① 鍼管　② 火傷　③ 透熱灸　④ 棒灸　⑤ 経穴　⑥ 線香　⑦ 専門学校

B 1. F   2. F   3. F

C 1. He invented an insertion tube.

2. The main difference between them is whether an insertion tube is used or not.

3. Kanshinho is.

APPENDIX

    4. They must study for three or four years.

    5. They put moxa on some acu-points on the patient's body and burn it in order to warm the body and cause a living body reaction

D 1. An acupuncturist puts a loquat leaf under moxa for preventing scar.

    2. It is acupuncture treatment that makes our low back pain relieve.

▶ Let's learn!　　p25

  ▶Exercise

  1. It was Tom's father who made this table and chair.

  2. It is tomorrow that Keiko will come back from Paris.

  3. It was a nice bag that my aunt sent me for my birthday.

CHAPTER 7　Needles for Treatment
治療で用いる鍼

NOTES　p28

A ① ステンレス　② ディスポーザブル　③ 感染　④ 細い　⑤ 太い　⑥ 松葉　⑦ 出血　⑧ 美容鍼灸

B 1. F　2. F　3. F

C 1. Needles for acupuncture are not hollow and get thinner to the point like pine needles. Needles for Western Medicine are hollow and cut sharply.

  2. They are made of Bianshi（砭石）.

  3. Needles for acupuncture are.

  4. It is because liquid can pass through.

  5. Thinner needles than hair are used.

D 1. Many German pediatricians are more and more interested in acupuncture today.

  2. Tom is kinder than any other student in the class.

▶ Let's learn!　　p29

  ▶Exercise

  1. 彼はますます背が高くなっています。

  2. チューリップは春になると、だんだん綺麗になります。

  3. 仕事を早く始めれば始めるほど、早く終わらせることができます。

  4. 運動をすればするほど、体重を減らすことができます。

CHAPTER 8 Acupuncture Treatment for Stiff Neck and Shoulder
肩こりの鍼治療

NOTES   p32

A ① 症候性肩こり ② ストレス ③ パソコン ④ VDT症候群 ⑤ 眼精疲労 ⑥ エアコン ⑦ 乳酸 ⑧ 血流

B 1. T 2. T 3. F

C 1. Soseki Natume did

2. A stressful life and the use of air conditioner do.

3. They are essential stiff shoulder, symptomatic stiff shoulder and psychogenic stiff shoulder.

D 1. One of my friends who has stiff neck and shoulder goes to the acupuncture clinic every week.

2. Ken bought the personal computer which was the cheapest at the store.

3. The man who is walking in the park is my father.

4. Mariko has a lot of friends who always help her.

5. The dress which she wore was wonderful.

▶ Let's learn!   p33

▶ Exercise

1. He cleans the new bike which was given for his birthday every day.

2. I like my cat whose name is MIMI.

3. The boy who is helping old people is the best student in the class.

4. Maggie showed the pictures which she took during the trip to Italy.

5. I learned flower arrangement from Ms. Ito, whose daughter is a famous dancer.

CHAPTER 9 Acupuncture Treatment for Pain
痛みに対する鍼治療

NOTES   p36

A ① 内因性オピオイド ② ナロキソン ③ ゲートコントロール理論 ④ アデノシン ⑤ 中枢性 ⑥ 末梢性

B 1. T 2. F 3. T

C 1. It is used as anesthesia.

2. It is a chemical subject which may reduce pain.

3. It demonstrated the other mechanism about painkilling caused by acupuncture treatment.

4. It is Ashisanri (ST36).

5. It is applied for twenty minutes.

D 1. Aspirin has been used as the medicine for headache for more than 100 years.

2. I have been to America many times but I have never been to Africa.

3. My mother has got acupuncture treatment since she was young.

▶ Let's learn!   p37

▶ Exercise

1. This car has been used by Ken.

2. The work has been done completely by Yumi.

3. John Lennon has been known all over the world.

CHAPTER 10   Sports Acupuncture
スポーツ鍼灸

📓 NOTES   p40

A ① コンディション　② 筋弛緩　③ 円皮鍼　④ パフォーマンス　⑤ 遅発性筋痛　⑥ 筋血流　⑦ マッサージ

B 1. F   2. T   3. F

C 1. They are pre-competition, intra-competition, and post –competition.

2. It is regulating athletes' body condition.

3. It is done for healing an athlete's body.

D 1. My purpose of traveling is to experience many things.

2. The man walking with a dog in the park is my uncle.

3. A friend of mine is traveling in the world treating patients with acupucnture.

▶ Let's learn!   p41

▶ Exercise

1. 私の父は私の誕生日にイタリア製のハンドバッグをくれました。

2. 2012年に建て替えられた東京駅は世界で最も美しい駅の一つです。

3. 多くの患者の慢性疾患を治療している鍼灸師はいつも一生懸命に働き、誰からも尊敬されています。

CHAPTER 11   Cosmetic Acupuncture
美容鍼灸

📓 NOTES   p44

A ① しわ　② 目の下のくま　③ 容姿　④ 血流　⑤ 肺　⑥ 脾　⑦ 安全性

B 1. F   2. F   3. T

C 1. The effect is anti-aging, such as making the face smaller, improving alopecia and losing weight.

2. No, it isn't. Cosmetic acupuncture targets the face, improving her or his appearance.

3. It is said that lung disorder, the weakness of the spleen and excessive drinking cause the facial wrinkles and pigmentations by the theory of Oriental Medicine.

4. Thinner needles are used.

5. No, it isn't.

D 1. Ken and John went to the library to study anatomy.

2. I am happy to have many friends to talk with.

3. Mariko studies cosmetic acupuncture and hopes to remove women's wrinkles in the future.

▶ Let's learn!   p45

▶Exercise

1. 私は重要な客を出迎えるために駅に行きました。(副詞用法で目的を示す)

2. ケイは腰痛治療のためのよいクリニックを探した。〈形容詞用法〉

3. メイは将来、東洋医学の専門家になりたい。(名詞用法)

4. ケイが東洋医学を習得することは重要です。(名詞用法)

CHAPTER 12   Kampo Medicine I
漢方薬 I

■ Notes   p49

A ① 薬味　② 薬性　③ 補瀉　④ 小柴胡湯　⑤ 同病異治　⑥ 白内障　⑦ 異病同治

B 1. F　2. T　3. T　4. T　5. F

C 1. The medicine utilized with herbs in China is referred to as Traditional Chinese Medicine.

The medicine used with herbs in Japan is referred to as Kampo Medicine.

2. It means treating a kind of illness by a different medicine.

3. It means treating different illness by a kind of medicine.

4. Japanese envoys to Sui China and to Tang China did.

D 1. I was prescribed Kampo Medicine to cure a cold.

2. Mr. Tanaka was given a watch for his birthday.

3. Tom has had low back pain treated with acupuncture.

▶ Let's learn!   p50

▶Exercise

1. A letter was written in Chinese by Ken.

2. The person is known well to them all.

3. Our cat was named MIMI (by us).

4. A special drink was made for Tom by Yoko.

5. The patient was given herbal medicine for a cold by the doctor.

Herbal medicine for a cold was given (to) the patient by the doctor.

CHAPTER 13 Kampo Medicine II
漢方薬 II

NOTES　p53

A　① 標治　② 本治　③④ 胃腸障害、婦人科疾患（順不同）　⑤ 気管支炎　⑥ 体質　⑦ 悪性腫瘍　⑧ 急性腎不全　⑨ 糖尿病　⑩ 運動療法

B　1. F　2. T　3. F

C　1. Honchi treatment is fundamental treatment : a physician improves the patient's constitution and removes a cause of illness.
Hyochi treatment is targeted treatment : a physician gets rid of the patient's symptom.
2. They are stomach and intestine disorders, chronic hepatitis, allergic diseases, mental disorders, gynecological diseases and cold.
3. They are myocardial infarction, cardiovascular diseases, high blood pressure, diabetes, malignant tumors and acute renal failure.
4. It is why Kampo Medicine is prescribed keeping specific remarks such as each patient's constitution, symptoms, and the progress of disease in mind.
5. No, it isn't.

D　1. It goes without saying that Oriental Medicine is difficult.
2. It is no use regretting having missed the train.

▶ **Let's learn!**　p54

▶ **Exercise**

> 上記動名詞の慣用表現を使用した英文を4文作ってください。
> 解答略

CHAPTER 14 Herbal Cuisine
薬　膳

NOTES　p56

A　① 中国伝統医学　② 食養　③ 食療　④ 陰陽　⑤ 体の状態　⑥ 未病　⑦ 食物繊維　⑧ いちじく　⑨ うり　⑩ 生姜

B　1. F　2. F　3. F

C　1. It is the theory of Traditional Chinese Medicine.
2. One is the therapeutic foods called "Shoku-yo" in Japanese, the other is the curing foods called "Shoku-ryo" in Japanese.
3. Because it includes much fiber.
4. It causes illness.
5. It is the body condition between health and disease.

D 1. You should drink a glass of water every morning.

2. Keiko can cook a delicious herbal cuisine.

3. According to the theory of TCM, it is thought that an eggplant and squash are effective for urinating.

▶ Let's learn!　　p57

　▶Exercise

1. 彼らは肥満を予防するためにもっと運動をするべきです。
2. 私たちは、いつでも高齢者に対し親切にするべきです。
3. あなたは東洋医学だけではなく西洋医学も勉強しなければなりません。
4. 私の友達はパーティーに間に合うのかしら。
5. 君たちは病院で大きな声で話してはいけません。

CHAPTER 15　Acupuncture Treatment in Foreign Countries
海外における鍼灸事情

NOTES　　p63

A ① 49　② 160　③ 虫垂炎除去手術　④ 麻薬中毒者　⑤ ハイルプラクティカー　⑥ 助産師　⑦ 開業　⑧ 鍼管無し

B 1. F　2. F　3. T

C 1. He or she is called Heilpraktiker in Germany.

2. They use needles without inserting tubes.

3. It means "in addition to Western Medicine".

4. Because they got the news about acupuncture treatment.

5. They study acupuncture and Chinese herb medicine.

D 1. More and more Americans are interested in acupuncture treatment.

2. We never forget the day when Great East Japan Earthquake occured.

3. It is my mother who made that delicious cake.

▶ Let's learn!　　p64

　▶Exercise

1. 彼は私に彼が以前住んでいた町のことについて話してくれた。
2. この時期、君たちは一生懸命勉強するべきです。
3. 彼があんなに怒った理由を知りたい。
4. このように鍼灸師は患者を治療する。

Grammar/Exercise
英文法・練習問題

受動態 p67 ▶Exercise

A 1. My work has not been finished yet.
2. This room must be kept clean all the time.
3. The person is known well to all of them.
4. His companions could not be kept up with by Oates.
5. Is that difficult problem being solved now ?
6. A new computer will be bought by my father tomorrow.
7. The injured is being carried to the hospital.
8. Our cat was named MIMI.
9. Who was that beautiful house built by ?
   By whom was that beautiful house built ?
10. They gave the patient much medicine to get well at the hospital.

B 1. with 2. in 3. of 4. with 5. in (by) 6. into 7. with 8. in 9. with 10. from

C 1. My younger brother was hit by the car and carried to the hospital at once.
2. He was taken care of by a nurse well during hospitalization.
3. I was very satisfied with the necklace which my father gave me for my birthday.

注意すべき受動態 p68 ▶Exercise

A 1. He was seen to take the purse by someone.
2. I will have my chair repaired by John.
3. The dog was made to sit quietly before eating.
4. Tom couldn't be caught up with by me.
5. That teacher is always spoken well of by students.

B 1. "Romeo and Juliet" is a Shakespeare's tragedy which is known well to everyone.
2. I bought a pretty hat made of wool at Kyoto station yesterday.

英文の時制 I p69 ▶Exercise

A 1. was reading 2. lost, saw 3. are 4. have been cleaning 5. have passed, left
6. will be traveling 7. is 8. has known 9. had been 10. will visit, hear

B 1. I am sure that you will progress in English if you study following the method I tell you.

解 答

英文の時制 Ⅱ　p70　▶Exercise

A 1. 彼らは来月で6年間あの橋を建設し続けている。
2. 彼は10年間彼女のことを知っていて、結婚した。
3. あなたは間違えられたかもしれないと思ったことがありますか？
4. 彼らが彼女を笑ったとき、彼女は怒らずにはいられなかった。
5. 彼はいつ日本に帰ってくるのかしら。

B 1. You will catch the 12 o'clock Nozomi if you leave now.
2. As I have never climbed Mt. Fuji, I will climb it this summer.
3. My younger brother came back to Japan from America last year.
   He seems to have had a hard time for getting accustomed to Japanese system as a pharmacist through a year because he had worked in America for fifteen years.

比　較　p71　▶Exercise

A 1. as, as, ever　2. more, important　3. no, more, than　4. no, less, than　5. the, better
6. better, than, to　7. superior　8. so, much, as　9. as, as, can　10. the ,most, of

B 1. She has <u>not less than</u> three good friends in Japan and two in America.
　　　　　　　（少なくとも）

関係代名詞　p73　▶Exercise

A 1. whose　2. what　3. which　4. which　5. which　6. what　7. that　8. whom　9. what
10. that

B 1. He missed the bus this morning, and what was worse, he left his homework at home.
2. What he likes the best is to travel abroad with friends.
3. They say the children who don't have breakfast lose their concentration in the class.

分　詞　p74　▶Exercise

A 1. repaired　2. traveling　3. made　4. satisfied　5. spoken　6. studying　7. injured
8. reading　9. understood　10. waiting

B 1. I saw Susan doing sunbathing in the park.
2. She bought a bag made in Japan in Italy.
3. The man fishing in the river is my uncle. I expect he will bring fresh fish to my house this evening.

不定詞　p75　▶Exercise

A 1. この本は難しすぎて私は読むことができません。
2. 彼は素敵な庭つきの家を買えるほど金持ちではありません。

87

APPENDIX

　　3. 私達は最終バスに間に合うように早く走った。

B 1. Yesterday I happened to ride on the same train that Tom did.

　　2. That Mathematics problem was too difficult for everybody to solve.

■ 助動詞　p76　　▶Exercise

A 1. must　2. cannot　3. should　4. would　5. must

B 1. I was surprised that he agreed with your opinion.

　　2. Mary's mother must have been beautiful when she was young.

東洋医学で英語を学ぶ
Medical English for Oriental Medicine　　ISBN978-4-263-24054-0

2013年3月25日　第1版第1刷発行
2020年5月25日　第1版第4刷発行

著者　高　木　久　代
　　　木　村　研　一
　　　西　村　甲
　　　高　木　健

発行者　白　石　泰　夫

発行所　医歯薬出版株式会社
〒113-8612　東京都文京区本駒込1-7-10
TEL.(03)5395-7641(編集)・7616(販売)
FAX.(03)5395-7624(編集)・8563(販売)
https://www.ishiyaku.co.jp/
郵便振替番号　00190-5-13816

乱丁，落丁の際はお取り替えいたします．　　印刷・真興社／製本・愛千製本所
© Ishiyaku Publishers, Inc., 2013.　Printed in Japan

本書の複製権・翻訳権・翻案権・上映権・譲渡権・貸与権・公衆送信権(送信可能化権を含む)・口述権は，医歯薬出版(株)が保有します．
本書を無断で複製する行為(コピー，スキャン，デジタルデータ化など)は，「私的使用のための複製」などの著作権法上の限られた例外を除き禁じられています．また私的使用に該当する場合であっても，請負業者等の第三者に依頼し上記の行為を行うことは違法となります．

[JCOPY] <出版者著作権管理機構　委託出版物>
本書をコピーやスキャン等により複製される場合は，そのつど事前に出版者著作権管理機構(電話03-5244-5088, FAX 03-5244-5089, e-mail:info@jcopy.or.jp)の許諾を得てください．

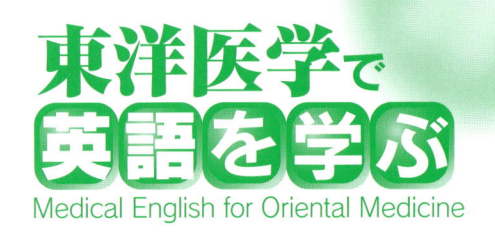

東洋医学で
英語を学ぶ
Medical English for Oriental Medicine